Ahead of the Curve

Lessons Learned from the Pandemic and How They Help Us Achieve Health and Happiness

By Mabel Hsin, M.D.

I would like to dedicate this book to my amazing husband Tony and daughters Alexis and Sydney, who help me appreciate the important things in life.

Table of Contents

Introduction i
Prologue: Three Pillars of Optimal Health vii
Reflection 1: Fragile to Agile 1
Reflection 2: KISS Away Diseases 14
Reflection 3: It's Not Me, It's You 26
Reflection 4: Killing it with Kindness 37
Reflection 5: Some of Us Are in This Together 44
Reflection 6: Hazards of Infodemic and the Dark Side of Hope 54
Reflection 7: I Can't Believe Me 68
Reflection 8: Collateral Damage and Safetyism 78
Reflection 9: Shooting Myself with Two Arrows 93
Reflection 10: My Own Reflection 105
Epilogue 108
Suggested Readings 110
Acknowledgments 111
About the Author 112

Introduction

It is July 2020, and I am getting bored out of my mind from just seeing people in my social bubble of 10, no offense to them. The swimming pools are still closed, along with my gym. So, I decided to pay a visit to my "BC" (Before COVID) self from December 2019 for a chat.

> BC (Before COVID) me: What's going on here? Are you a twin sister I never knew I had?

> AC (After COVID) me: I'm your future self, here for a brief visit from the summer of 2020. I came to give you some essential tips about how you can stay ahead of the curve.

> BC: Stay ahead of what curve? What does that even mean?

AC: The Pandemic curve. There is a virus pandemic starting within the month. It's from a novel virus called COVID-19. You'll be hearing a lot about it soon. It will dominate all the media and headlines for the foreseeable future. People will stop caring about what the Kardashians are doing and even less about what they are wearing.

You'll hear phrases like "flattening the curve," "peak of the curve," and "ahead of the curve." This refers to the importance of slowing down the pandemic before the infection rate becomes dangerously rampant and difficult to control. Once it is widespread in the community, it becomes increasingly difficult (if not impossible) to control.

BC: It's hard to believe this is really going to happen. A full-on pandemic. Incredible. As physicians, we knew that this was a real possibility. We know that staying ahead of the curve applies not only to the pandemic but also to our personal wellbeing. So many aspects of our wellness hinge on us practicing healthy habits, both mentally and physically, so we don't end up with conditions like dementia, depression, anxiety disorder, addictions, diabetes, heart disease, cancer...I can go on and on. These are all potentially preventable conditions.

AC: Exactly. During the pandemic, some countries will manage to stay ahead of the curve, while others will fall behind. This will have huge consequences on how the countries will fare, both in the health of their populations as well as their economies. This pandemic will be an opportunity to teach us that everything can change in an instant.

BC: How will this impact my family and me? I have work plans lined up all year. I have vacation plans for the summer. I'm starting to look for flights to Europe.

AC: Don't plan any trips and cancel all flights for next year! While you are at it, you might want to change your investments from high risk to guaranteed savings. The markets are in for a wicked roller coaster ride! Oh, and stock up on some toilet paper.

BC: This is a nightmare. I'm going to wake up any second, right?

AC: Listen to me. This is serious. All those things you took for granted, like vacations, work, and seeing your friends-- enjoy them now, because they will all disappear next year.

You live for the future, thinking, "When I get my raise, or when I have some free time, I'll be happier." When that future you are planning for is taken away, you will be left with nothing. Live each day as a gift, and you will enjoy many gifts.

Instead of vacationing to Europe, let me take you through a journey of self-discovery to help you achieve well-being physically, mentally, and spiritually.

BC: Did you say you are taking me on a trip? This sounds like a lot of magical thinking. You know, with my medical background, I'm not into magical thinking.

AC: Rest assured, so am I. I am you, remember? The information I'm going to tell you is all based on science and research. It's the truth as we know it in July 2020.

BC: I do love the scientific process and evidence-based information.

AC: One of the first things I want to tell you is that we need to be students. We need to learn from countries that will be successful in controlling the pandemic and apply their strategies. We need to observe countries that will fail and avoid those actions that will lead to their failures during the first phase of the pandemic. In the same way, we can study wisdom from the many philosophers before us and use them to enrich our lives.

There are lessons we can learn from the leaders who will put their countries ahead of the curve during the pandemic. I will detail their skills and attributes and give you action plans to build them yourself. By investing in yourself, you will not only become a better human being, but you will also become a happier and more resilient leader. There isn't any magic to building these skills and attributes. The strategies and assignments I provide will require a concerted effort, practice, and consistency.

BC: I'm crazy busy, putting in 60 to 70 hours at work. I don't have time for this.

AC: Working on developing these attributes does not take time. It *gives* time. Numerous studies show that when your physical and mental health improves, you'll have more energy and mental resources, allowing you to be more productive.

BC: So how am I supposed to learn from this pandemic?

AC: From a pandemic perspective, we can learn in two ways: from seeing what other countries did wrong and avoiding their mistakes or learning what other countries did right and modeling their strategies.

From an individual perspective, we can take the same approach. In the past, psychology was about learning what is wrong with people. That has been found to be helpful in trying to find solutions to get patients back to wellness when they are ill.

However, thanks to the pioneer of Positive Psychology Martin Seligman, we are learning what is right with people and discovering how we can flourish and find contentment. This latter approach has allowed us to discover how we can thrive as human beings. Much of this has been known and taught for centuries by philosophers like Socrates, Plato, and Aristotle. But we now have the science to prove that attributes like kindness, gratitude, altruism, and a sense of purpose, really do make people happier and more content.

Here is how this journey works.

There will be nine reflections I will take you through. You'll develop the tenth piece of learning on your own.

Each reflection starts with available data during the summer of 2020 on the COVID-19 pandemic and how it applies to a society or country. I will take the lesson learned from the pandemic and guide you on how to develop the skills we learn from the lesson to strengthen and enrich you mentally, physically, and or spiritually.

A series of questions will be posed for you because we learn about ourselves through deep reflection. If you are to be truly honest with yourself, some of the questions posed in the reflections should make you feel uncomfortable. Truth is often uncomfortable, but facing and confronting discomfort is how we grow.

An action plan will be offered. These will be proven strategies to help you thrive and increase your resilience. It is your responsibility to take action. You need to commit to completing each lesson plan. *Knowing does not equal doing.*

Finally, for ease of reference for you to activate your action plan, you can download a PDF from **DrMabelHsin.ca/action-plan** and fill in your exercises. We all know what we should do. The action plan is there to help you do it.

In everything you do in life, you get out what you put in, whether it's learning a new language, sport, music instrument, or school courses. The same applies here. If you want to flourish, you need to adapt to change. And trust me, the changes you are about to witness are so monumental you cannot imagine.

Many of the patient stories in this book come from my 30 years of clinical experience. To protect their privacy, their names and some details have been changed. Please note that any patient stories described in this book are a way to express the flaws and fortitudes that exist in each of us. These stories help us recognize our own strengths and weaknesses.

Prologue: Three Pillars of Optimal Health

Before I embark on the reflections, I would first like to explain to you the Three Pillars of Optimal Health. These are what I consider to be the habits we must adopt to transform our lives to become the best version of ourselves mentally, physically, and spiritually. You will hear me refer to these Three Pillars throughout the reflections.

The Three Pillars are:

Exercise

Mindfulness practice

Social connection

Let me briefly explain why these are the foundations to becoming an awesome you.

Exercise

The human body is made to move. Exercise is not only good for our body physically but also mentally. Exercise is as effective as medications for anxiety and depression, without the risk of side effects. It is far better than medications for improving our sleep. It is better than caffeine for increasing our energy. When we move, our brain produces all sorts of wonderful neurotransmitters and neurohormones that make us think better and reduce our risk of dementia. Best of all, exercise does not mean you need to spend money on a gym membership. It can be as simple as a brisk daily walk

Mindfulness Practice

How would you like to be fifty years old but have the wisdom of a sage and the mental processing power of a twenty-year-old? Well, those are the implications of results from scientific studies on mindfulness.

Mindfulness is about bringing moment to moment awareness to our thoughts and emotions without judgment, so we can respond wisely to situations.

Mindfulness is now part of mainstream science. It is no longer just voodoo magic practised by new-age hippies. It is practised by astronauts and elite athletes. Mindfulness programs are used in training for Navy Seals, law enforcement personnel, firefighters, and medical students across North America.

Mindfulness practice is still relatively new for many people. It is a crucial pillar because it not only has numerous benefits for our wellbeing (as backed up by thousands of studies in the past decades), but it also helps us overcome the mental barriers that may divert us from implementing the other two pillars.

Many people think of mindfulness as simply meditation. But it is much more than that. Meditation is the formal part of mindfulness practice. I see meditation as a conduit to help us achieve mindfulness.

There are numerous research data, including MRIs and EEGs, showing how mindfulness practice can bring tremendous changes to our brains via new cell growth and connections, something called neuroplasticity. These changes allow us to be calmer, to act more wisely, and with more compassion. Not only that, but there is also abundant evidence showing it can actually slow down the aging effects on the brain and cells in our bodies. As a bonus, people who practise mindfulness have superior immune systems, which can prevent or help fight off infections more efficiently. Mindfulness is like a natural, safe vaccine against infections.

Social Connection

Did you wonder why I put social connection as my third Pillar of Optimal Health rather than healthy eating? Here's something that may blow your mind. Studies show that social connection has a far greater impact on our wellbeing than healthy eating. Humans are social creatures. Connecting with people, we appreciate socially increases wonderful feel-good hormones like oxytocin and lowers our stress hormones like cortisol. Furthermore, it energizes us, reduces our ruminations and negative thinking, and increases our self-esteem. It also increases our prosocial behaviours, which is simply a fancy way of saying it makes us nicer and kinder.

Healthy Eating

Okay, even though healthy eating did not quite make it to my top Three Pillars, it is still an important aspect of our health, so here's my two cents on the topic.

Which is the best diet? Is it high fat ketogenic, intermittent fasting, low carb, vegetarian, vegan, or gluten-free? There are probably more diets to choose from than shoes in Kylie Jenner's closet.

Numerous scientists argue over which diet is superior. Their data often contradict each other. Are they all wrong? Perhaps the better explanation is that the ideal diet depends on the individual. Here's the one consistent thing in nutrition research: human beings living on planet earth should eat *real* food. People want experts to tell them exactly what and how to eat. They make eating into a complicated and mystifying production. The fact is healthy eating is a simple concept. Minimize processed or artificially prepared foods and enjoy a variety of goodies that nature offers us. Michael Pollan, who has written several books on the subject, summarizes his advice on food in seven simple words: "Eat food, not too much, mostly plants."

So there you are, the Three Pillars of Optimal Health.

Now let's see what lessons we can learn from the COVID-19 Pandemic to help us build Hope, Health, and Happiness.

Reflection 1: Fragile to Agile

"Prevention is so much better than healing because it saves the labor of being sick." ~Albert Einstein

---

Lesson from COVID-19

> BC: No doubt you have a lot to share about the pandemic. Where do we begin?

> AC: Let me begin by explaining how this pandemic is not a Black Swan event as some people implied.

> BC: A Black Swan event? What is that exactly?

> AC: According to Nassim Taleb's definition: a "Black Swan phenomenon" is rare, high profile, and unexpected; it has tremendous impact, and in hindsight, it could have been predicted. Black Swan events will decimate systems that are fragile. I will explain how to overcome this fragility later.

> BC: Hang on, haven't scientists and doctors been warning for many years that we are due for an impending pandemic?

> AC: Precisely. That's why this is a White Swan event, which is an event that is devastating but completely predictable. What will be unpredictable is the devastation it will cause to the global economy and how unprepared many countries will be, *despite* the many warnings from scientists and doctors.

On January 4, 2020, with a single tweet, the world will be put on notice. A cluster of pneumonia cases will be reported in Wuhan, China, with their causes unknown.

When COVID-19 arrives, it will not be immediately clear whether this was, in fact, the "big event" that epidemiologists had been warning about for decades or just another novel virus that would not significantly impact the world.

With this hindsight, we can look back and see that every country will be at a similar risk with the virus. Some agile countries will be able to adapt and manage the crisis quite effectively, while the fragile countries will experience devastation.

Countries that will do well are those that are prepared for the pandemic and will have taken many similar actions:

They will have the capacity in the hospitals.

They will have coordinated efforts right from the start.

They will be decisive on immediately implementing things like aggressive contact tracing and coordinated testing

They will have consistent messaging that provided clear guidance to their citizens.

Countries that will do poorly will ignore the issue until things explode.

Instead of putting out the fire while it is smouldering, the unsuccessful countries will wait until the fire is out of control.

MERS, also known as Middle East Respiratory Syndrome, was another coronavirus outbreak that started in the Arabian Peninsula in 2012, with a death rate of 30-40%. It was brought to South Korea in 2015 from a traveller returning from the Middle East. After experiencing MERS, South Korea had ramped up their pandemic preparation between 2015 and 2020, so they will be ready when the COVID-19 pandemic hits. Countries like South Korea and Singapore that were prepared before the pandemic will be able to shut down quickly despite their dense populations. They will do aggressive testing and contact tracing right from the start. Other countries will be trying desperately to ramp up their measures in the midst of the pandemic.

The benefits of these preventative measures will become obvious when the well-prepared countries are able to come out of population lockdown well before the unsuccessful countries, sparing them severe damage to the health of their population and their economies as of phase one of the pandemic.

How we can stay ahead of the curve and protect our own health by turning fragile to agile

Countries that are prepared in advance will be much less fragile than others that will not be as prepared. They will have the agility to move quickly to contain the outbreak because they will be ready for such an event. For our personal wellbeing, we can learn from the mistakes made by the countries that make them fragile: ignoring the warnings, not being prepared, not acting on the problem until it is too late. We can also learn from the countries that will do well during the pandemic. These agile countries will be resilient because they will have measures put in place to prevent devastating outcomes.

This is the first lesson in getting ahead of the curve.

Can we avoid our own personal Black Swan event? Can we prepare ourselves so that we can be agile instead of fragile if we were to face a devastating event, like contracting the COVID-19 infection, or predictable diseases like diabetes and heart disease? Can we develop resiliency mentally and physically so that we can prevent some diseases altogether, like many types of cancers? The answer is a resounding yes. Prevention is always the best defense.

Conditions like Type 2 diabetes, obesity, and many cancers, while they are often not Black Swan phenomena, still have devastating effects on our health. These conditions are not rare, and most are predictable and preventable. So why do patients often react with such surprise (as if it is a Black Swan phenomenon) when given these diagnoses?

These are conditions that are within our power to prevent. However, like countries that will be prepared for the pandemic, we must also be prepared for these conditions. We must and can prevent them through the Three Pillars of Optimal Health introduced earlier: Exercise, Mindfulness training, and Social Connection.

To Turn Fragile into Agile

According to Nassim Taleb, we can turn the fragile systems into antifragile. He describes antifragile as an ability to thrive from stress. One way to increase antifragility is by introducing redundancy. He was describing antifragility as a mathematical idea to be used in risk analysis. However, I feel the same concepts can be applied to human behaviours.

For our personal wellbeing, we can think of the opposite of fragile as agile: an ability to adapt to changes and stressors. Darwin did not, in fact, say "survival of the fittest" but rather survival of the most adaptable: "It is not the strongest of the species that survive, nor the most intelligent. It is the one that is most adaptable to change." We can turn our body and mind into an agile system that can adapt easily and prevent diseases that are predictable. By being agile, we can also adapt with ease to negative conditions and events that befall us, such as job and family stressors. Just like the predictability of the pandemic, when we recognize the possibility of a negative event, we can prepare for it. If we are prepared for the possible diseases and difficulties that can transpire, we can either avoid it or mitigate its damages.

The human body already has this redundancy built-in. We have two kidneys, so if one fails, there is another one. We have two lungs, so if one collapses, we have another. The redundancy in the case for turning fragile to agile means not just eating better, but also other measures like exercising and training our brains to think and reason through learning and critical thinking, rather than just taking in whatever sensational headlines tell us. We can also train our brains to become less reactive, to be calmer. In doing this, we reduce our level of negative stress, which can ravage our physical and mental health. We nourish our body, mind, and spirit. This is the foundation of the Three Pillars of Optimal Health.

When we don't practice the Three Pillars of Optimal Health, we become fragile. We become susceptible to diseases and illnesses. But when we practice the Three Pillars regularly, we stay ahead of the curve.

Exercise and healthy eating have been promoted as a good lifestyle choice for a very long time. If you were to only focus on exercise, connecting with people you like, and diet, you would become less fragile but would still be missing a key pillar. Mindfulness practice will help us go from fragile to agile. It increases our resiliency mentally and physically. The Three Pillars will help us take care of our body and mind in good times, nurture them, and allow them to function at peak performance level, so it has the power to overcome difficulties.

This is the same reason we train our firefighters when there is no fire. Redundancy is built into their training. They receive instructions not only on how to put out fires but also on understanding building structures, first aid, movement of gases, and so on. The day that there is a fire, they are ready. They have built agility through their training to be able to adapt to different situations, making them more resilient to disasters. This is a far better strategy than waiting until they are in the midst of a burning building before teaching them what to do.

If the measures are so simple, why do many people struggle to go from having the desire to act and actually taking action? One of the first things we need to do to start building agility is to identify and overcome the common barriers that prevent us from acting.

Barrier 1: The Instant Gratification Trap

The first step most people need to take is to overcome instant gratification. For example, having that extra scoop of ice cream is so much more instantly gratifying than being mindful about things we can do now to avoid diabetes five years down the road. Health is about avoiding bad habits now.

When we give in to instant gratification, pleasure is transient. Soon, you want more: more social media, junk food, TV. You are never satisfied. You adapt, and you end up needing more to feel satisfied. To get ahead of the curve and overcome our fragility, we need to break free from constantly seeking instant gratification. We will address how to do this in the action plans.

Barrier 2: The Genetics Rationalization Trap

Another thing I see with patients is that they sometimes give in to a victim-like mentality, in which they maintain the belief that they are genetically fated to have a negative health outcome. They create a hopelessness that holds them back from making the lifestyle changes. For example, they will believe that they are destined to become obese because their parents are overweight.

Sometimes a little scientific knowledge without context can be dangerous. While it is true that genetics do cause some diseases, that is not the whole story.

What most people do not realize is that our genetics do not determine our fate. Just because we carry the gene for certain conditions, environment and lifestyle choices play a tremendous role in whether these genes are turned on. This is the field of epigenetics, where our choices determine which genes are turned on or off.

Think about this for a moment: Our genes have remained the same in the past century. Why then has there been such a huge increase in obesity rates in the developed countries within the past few decades?

It is estimated that genetics contribute to about half of all obesity cases. That means the other half is from factors within our control. We also have much more control over our genetic risk of developing other conditions than we think, such as Type 2 diabetes, cardiovascular disease, and numerous cancers.

Similarly, many people feel hopeless and struggle with weight loss, not because they are lazy or weak-willed, but because they are focused on the wrong outcomes. Many will exercise regularly, eat a diet so healthy it would put a monk to shame, and yet remain unable to lose weight. Here is what I say to that.

Do not focus on the scale. Focus on the process. I will discuss this further in the next reflection.

To demonstrate these ideas, I would like to share with you a story of two patients.

Case Study 1 - Walter

The first patient, Walter, was a successful 48-year old man who founded a thriving business. He was always on the run and extremely busy. His lifestyle did not allow him to take care of his health and wellbeing. Despite my constant encouragement to adopt lifestyle strategies through better eating and exercise to control his diabetes, his reply was always the same. He did not have the time.

At the age of 67, when he retired from the company he had built, he was confined to a wheelchair with heart issues, back, hip, and knee issues, as well as vision issues. He was not able to enjoy his retirement because he spent it going to doctors' appointments and undergoing tests to keep him alive. Sadly, there are so many Walters out there.

Case Study 2 - Mike

Contrast that with Mike. He is an enthusiastic young man, highly intelligent, and believes in becoming the best version of himself. His enthusiasm for life is palpable when he walks into a room. Both his parents were quite obese and sedentary. Rather than sitting back and allowing fate to dictate his weight, he empowered himself by regularly exercising and eating healthy since he was a teen. He became a fit athlete, playing in varsity sports teams while attending university. Despite his genetic disposition for obesity from both parents, he paved his own path through positive lifestyle habits.

Mike may never see a Black Swan event related to his health because of the steps he has taken to get ahead of the curve. If he does have a major incident, his positive lifestyle habits make him agile, which will put him in a much better position to have a successful outcome. Meanwhile, Walter's life has been destroyed by his personal White Swan: his complications from many years of uncontrolled diabetes were devastating and predictable.

The key lesson in this is that we each have a choice about which path we are going to follow. Since you are reading this book, it seems like you are ready to follow Mike's path. Congratulations!

The first action you need to take is to put aside all the excuses to not start working on the Three Pillars of Optimal Health and take action to begin reducing your fragility and increase your agility.

Excuses are the biggest barriers to our success.

I know what you are thinking: "Can't you come up with strategies that are more exciting than just telling me to exercise more, connect with good people, and train my brain? What happened to the latest miracle diet or supplement?"

These measures I am talking about are neither flashy nor trendy. This is why so many people ignore them. Yes, people want miracles. But asking for miracles is as useful as offering stilettos to marathon runners.

However, if you stick around and follow along with the lessons I lay out, I will unveil the one key that can unlock all the abilities to achieve these strategies.

Questions to Ponder

Here are some questions I'd like you to consider. It's especially important for you not to just think of the answers in your head but to actually write them down. When you put them down in concrete words, the concepts become much better integrated into your mind. It helps to clarify your thoughts and increases purposefulness. Remember, all these questions and action plans can be downloaded from DrMabelHsin.com

What changes do I need to make to take care of my future self?

_____

_____

_____

What habits do I have that are not serving me well?

_____

_____

_____

Why do I persist in these habits? Is it for instant gratification? Will that short-term pleasure be worth it?

_____

_____

_____

What would my future self say to my present self about these habits?

_____

_____

_____

Turbo-charge Tip #1

Want to turbo-charge the insight you can attain from this exercise? Let the questions and answers percolate for a few days in your subconscious mind. Then come back to the questions and explore the answers again. You can do this with all the question sections in each reflection.

Action Plan

Habits I want to adopt:

_____

_____

_____

My motivation for adopting these habits:

_____

_____

_____

My intrinsic value for wanting to adopt these habits:

_____

_____

_____

Note: intrinsic values are values that are for your own sake, not for the sake of something else. When you act according to your intrinsic values, there is greater contentment and chance of success.

For example, what is the reason you want to lose weight? So you can be healthier? Feel better? Enjoy lifting your grandchild when you retire? These are intrinsic values.

However, if you want to lose twenty pounds so you can fit into that dress to impress people at your friend's wedding, that's extrinsic value. What happens after the wedding when you no longer need to impress everyone else?

This is going to take a lot of reflection. The answers can feel uncomfortable, especially if you are honest with yourself. Embrace the discomfort. It is a catalyst for growth.

Reflection 2: KISS Away Diseases

"The secret of getting ahead is getting started." ~Mark Twain

Lesson from COVID-19

> BC: Will it be a revolutionary vaccine or drug that will control the pandemic?

> AC: During the crisis, people are all looking at, and anxiously waiting for dubious "cures" or a blockbuster drug like the drug hydroxychloroquine. Many will form unrealistic expectations like vaccines availability by summer of 2020. None of this panned out to be true during the first phase of the pandemic.

> BC: What will be found to be effective against the virus?

> AC: The KISS principle: Keep It Simple Silly. Simple measures like hand washing and physical distancing. This is the reason scientists repeatedly stress the importance of behavioural change to control the virus.

From Public Health's point of view, it will be meticulous contact tracing and quarantine of those infected. Another measure important in the early stage of a pandemic is having enough stockpiles of PPE and supply chains. All of which are low tech strategies. Not very glamorous, but certainly tried and true measures.

I am all for innovation and technology. It has saved so many lives and made our day to day activities far easier, from ventilators to washing machines and microwave ovens.

Technology does not mean we should abandon the basic simple and effective interventions that are available to everyone. We have an exaggerated reliance on the power of technology. Some of the most basic interventions turned out to be the most effective.

There will be an interesting story in May, two months after the lockdown. Ontario numbers will not come down for several reasons. During his insanely busy workdays looking after sick patients in the hospital, a Toronto infectious disease specialist will take it upon himself to put into Google maps addresses of infected patients that come through the hospital. By doing this simple action, he will discover where infection clusters were. He will mobilize targeted testing in that area, which will uncover a number of infected cases that may have gone undetected.

Rather than relying on the existing testing measures from the government, as it was clearly not effective at that time, he will take up the responsibility himself to discover where the cases were. No fancy new tracing technology will be used. Just simply entering addresses into Google maps.

We have more control than we think. Sometimes we cannot sit back and wait for someone else to look after our problems. Sometimes we need to take responsibility ourselves. And the solutions are often simpler than we think.

KISS and Our Physical Health

Most people know about Type 1 and Type 2 diabetes. I'm going to share with you a little-known fact. There is a type 3 diabetes.

Type 3 Diabetes

Type 1 diabetes occurs in people who cannot produce any insulin. This is not related to any lifestyle habits. Type 2 occurs due to insulin resistance in the body. Type 2 diabetes is mostly related to obesity and lack of exercise, which is why it can be prevented or controlled through lifestyle habits.

Type 3 diabetes, on the other hand, is also known as Alzheimer's disease. It is from the effects of insulin resistance on the brain. When our waistline increases, our brain shrinks. This is one of the most devastating diseases that frightens most people. If you want to reduce your risk for Alzheimer's, you need to practice the Three Pillars.

Here is something most doctors know that patients do not. The medications we have presently for Alzheimer's are not highly effective. For decades, scientists have been working on creating a vaccine for Alzheimer's unsuccessfully. Exercise, on the other hand, is far more effective in reducing this debilitating condition than any medication we have. Exercise and mindfulness training are considered by neuroscientists to be *the* two most powerful interventions for brain health. This is the KISS principle, which helps us stay ahead of the curve.

To demonstrate the effectiveness of KISS and taking personal responsibility, I will share with you a story of two patients. At the end of these two case studies, I will pose a question for you.

Case Study 3 - Emily

Emily is twenty-four-years-old, tall, five foot nine, with a slim build. She does not like to cook, so she eats take-outs and processed foods most days. She does not exercise because she feels she is slim enough, so she doesn't see the point.

Case Study 4 - Marilyn

Marilyn is an upbeat and cheerful fifty-six-year-old mother of two grown sons. She has a short and stoutly built frame, weighing 165 pounds, at a height of five-foot-one inch. She works out three days per week with a personal trainer and walks another two days per week for exercise. She is careful with her diet, eating mostly salads and unprocessed foods. However, she was frustrated that her weight would not come down after an initial loss of twenty pounds, despite those consistent efforts for over six months.

Which of these two patients do you think had a fatty liver detected by ultrasound?

Drum roll, please...the answer is the first patient, Emily.

In North America, people tend to associate weight loss with physical appearance rather than health, which is why it was often difficult for me to convince my thin patients to exercise and eat healthily. Even though Emily appeared thin on the outside, an autopsy will reveal the results of her lifestyle on the inside.

Yes, it is possible to be overweight yet to be healthier than a skinny person.

Barriers to Weight Loss

Want to know the #1 solution to obesity? Prevention. Once a person gains weight, it is very difficult to lose it.

When people gain weight, the body sees the new weight as a new setpoint. Homeostasis refers to our bodies' ability to maintain a stable environment, be it our temperature, fluid content, or weight. This is like our home thermostat. Because of homeostasis, once someone loses weight, they need to exercise more to maintain weight loss as the body tends to want to go back to the previous set point. This is a great source of frustration for many people trying to lose weight. When despair and hopelessness set in, they give up the healthy behavioural changes in frustration, and they berate themselves for failing. Out of desperation, they turn to fad diets and supplements promising miracle weight loss. It seems like everyone, including their house cat, has a secret to weight loss. This results in their weight yo-yo-ing, which is even more detrimental to our health and aggravates the problem.

Just as we must learn to manage to live with COVID-19 because it will be with us for a long time, we must learn to manage obesity. Obesity is not a condition to be discriminated against or seen as a character weakness. It needs to be regarded as a chronic disease. Like any chronic disease, the behavioural changes required to manage it must be maintained.

With obesity, once further weight loss is unsuccessful, it is more useful to focus on healthy behaviours of simply maintaining the weight and preventing repeated weight gain. This focus will prevent despair of failure. And here is the good news. Even if that person remains overweight, the health risks for diabetes and cardiovascular disease is still decreased because of the improved lifestyle changes. For example, exercise reduces insulin resistance. It also helps us fight against our current epidemic of Type 3 diabetes.

Owning the Problem

I want to highlight another conversation I had with a different patient.

I pointed out gently to Jenny that she had gained 20 lbs since her last physical. Her response? "Yeah, I know. What are *you* going to do about it?" Jenny's first step to becoming successful in managing her weight is when she changes her response to "Yeah, I know. What can *I* do about it?"

Personally, I have no issues with my patients gaining excess weight—it happens. It is more important that they are aware if it impacts their health. If they are aware and recognize this, that means they can fix it and improve their health. But the first step is taking responsibility. Some estimate that 90% of our health has to do with what we do, not what our doctors do with us. As with technology, I am all for medication *if* used appropriately. But we have more control over our own health than we often realize.

The key to preventative health is behavioural change. Let us continue to use weight loss as an example, but keep in mind the same applies to other health habits you may be challenged with, like smoking cessation. The prefrontal cortex, otherwise known as our executive brain, does the planning, impulse control, and other wonderful functions. It is similar to executives in companies. It is rational and logical. Humans are supposed to have the most developed prefrontal cortex in the animal kingdom, although I often wonder about that after witnessing some of the behaviours in reality TV.

Much of our unhealthy eating is hedonic, which means we eat not because we are hungry, but for the dopamine fix, almost like an addiction. The one thing we have control over is our executive brain. To lose weight successfully, in addition to eating better, we also need to nourish our executive brain through the Three Pillars.

It is more effective to focus on behavioural changes rather than how much weight to lose. The journey is more important than the destination. Although it is okay to have a weight loss goal, it is more effective to focus on the habits of healthy eating rather than focusing on how much weight we want to lose. This is the journey.

Here is some great news which is hot off the press! In a paper that will be published in July 2020, Canadian Medical Association will publish new guidelines on obesity which define it not by the size of a person, but rather by whether a person's fat impairs their health. The new guidelines emphasize the focus on improving patients' health rather than simply losing weight.

The Miracle Traps

Patients often rely on others to "fix" their problems when the problem is in *their* power to "fix." We must stop looking at dubious claims out there on magical cures, promising life-changing miracles. The only things life-changing are things *you* do, and they are not quick fixes. There are no "hacks" in this path.

Throughout history, charlatans have been peddling snake oils as magic cures for everything our heart desires. Nowadays, they use pseudoscience to prey on people's vulnerabilities, of wanting to look younger, thinner, have more energy...

They use scientific language to make themselves sound credible. Some are so convincing that even professionals like doctors and nurses are fooled. It can be exceedingly difficult to separate fact from fiction. Unfortunately, in addition to wasting their money, some people have been physically harmed and even died from these magic potions. Rather than turning to miracles to grant us good health, we must recognize that often it is within our own powers to accomplish using KISS.

KISS away Sleep Deprivation

How often have you skipped out on sufficient sleep because you were too busy? Because sleep is so unproductive, right? We all fall into this trap. What disorders do you think are affected by lack of sleep?

Did you know that a lot of behavioural issues in ADHD kids are reduced once their sleep habits improve? Sleep deprivation increases anxiety, depression, and obesity, among other problems. Not to mention, it also decreases our productivity and increases our risk of Alzheimer's. The time you spend on getting enough sleep, you will gain back from an increase in productivity.

Many people depend on sleeping pills rather than personal practices to improve sleep, such as no screen time two hours before bed, exercise, and meditation. Technology cannot replace good habits. Sleeping pills are bad for our brains, and they also increase our risk of dementia. Again, we can prevent this with the simple principle of KISS instead of relying on pills.

With KISS, You Don't Need Willpower to Succeed

These solutions are incredibly simple and effective, so why is it so difficult for people to develop the discipline to follow through with the behavioural changes they know are important?

Relying on our existing willpower alone is highly ineffective. Willpower is a function of the executive brain. Our resource of willpower is limited. That is why people tend to take in most of their excess or unhealthy calories at night. We are too exhausted physically and mentally from making decisions all day to resist the temptations.

Let me show you how to overcome a lack of willpower so that you can employ the KISS principle rather than seeking miracle cures. Again, the solutions are simple.

Questions to Ponder

What areas am I relying on others on when I should be the one taking responsibility? (Is it a friend to start an exercise program? Someone to make me healthier meals?)

_____

_____

_____

What actions do I need to take to implement these lifestyle changes? (For example, to improve my sleep habits or eat better.)

_____

_____

_____

Turbocharge Tip #2

Here's another way to increase your insight into these self-reflective questions.

After recording your answers to each of the questions, ask yourself, "why." Ask why three times and record the answers. Again, you can do this with every question section in the book.

Action Plans

What do people need to do to affect the behavioural change?

Setting Goals

First, own it! You are the one responsible for what you do unless, of course, you are a celebrity. Only *you* are responsible for your well-being.

Decide what behavioural changes you want to make.

Make the goal small and attainable lest you set yourself up for failure.

Each time you reach that goal, move the goal post a little further. This will give you the motivation to persevere. Each time you reach a goal, you get a shot of dopamine, the neurotransmitter that motivates you to do things. Success begets success.

Okay, so now you are thinking: I thought you said to focus on the journey, not the goal? Yes, but that does not mean you do not set goals. Just do not get attached to them.

In setting goals with weight loss, for example, go with the 1% rule. Start with a goal of, say, 1% of your body weight. Once you achieve that, set the next goal at another 1%. That way, it is easier to reach the goal, and you feel rewarded whenever you do.

Implementation/Intention

How can we apply those concepts to weight loss and exercise so that we do not have to rely on our will power?

We can apply a technique called Implementation/Intention

As described by James Clear in *Atomic Habits*, you write down your Intention-- the habit you want to build. Then write down when and where.

Let's say you want to start an exercise program. You write down when you will exercise and where.

Here is the beauty of adopting these habits and the importance of the journey rather than the goal. Remember, even if you do not lose weight, as long as you are honest with yourself, the behavioural changes in adopting a healthier diet and increasing exercise will result in a healthier you.

WHEN				
WHERE				
INTENTION				

Reflection 3: It's Not Me, It's You

"We are what we repeatedly do; therefore, excellence is not an act but a habit." ~Aristotle

Lesson from COVID-19

AC: Early in the pandemic, mistakes will be made because of lack of information about the virus. Despite their best efforts and intentions, blunders will occur.

BC: It must be quite difficult making the right decisions since so little will be known about a new virus. How will various leaders respond to these oversights?

> AC: Despite these first missteps, some leaders will recognize their errors, take ownership of their mistakes, and put new measures into action to correct those mistakes. Despite being one of the countries that will fare the best, Singapore's prime minister Lee Hsien Loong for example, will announce that mistakes were made early on. He will name all the errors and vow to take corrective measures. The outcome? He will have the trust of the population resulting in remarkably high compliance rates with the policies. They will be able to turn around the infection rates and get things under control

To get ahead of the curve, when these leaders recognize the errors, they proceed to correct the course. Making mistakes is part of being human. The key is taking responsibility for the errors and making amends.

In contrast, there will be a lot of blaming and finger-pointing from some countries' leadership that did not handle the crisis well. They will make excuses for the poor outcomes in their countries. We will see countries try to explain their high death rates by saying, "we have a high population of elderly people." Yet, Japan will do extremely well, and they have one of the highest numbers of seniors in their population.

Others will claim they cannot contain the spread because of their high population density. However, places like Japan, Singapore, and South Korea all have extremely high-density populations, and yet they fared much better than other countries with low population density. When things are not going well, some politicians lash out and blame everyone else. And they're not the only people who like to redirect blame.

Why do people blame others?

Blaming means less work because we do not have to be held accountable. It makes people less vulnerable and distances them from being associated with mistakes. Blaming others during stressful times also gives people a sense of control and protects their ego. But a great leader takes ownership of their problems.

When we blame others, we lose the chance to learn and grow personally. It reduces our empathy for other people. Blaming is also contagious. When one person starts the blame game, others follow.

Good leadership is about effective action. Instead of sitting there looking for people to blame, good leaders take responsibility for their actions. They have a vision for success, and they give people compelling reasons to do the right things.

Stopping the blame game and taking responsibility in your life to stay ahead of the curve

Let me share a story with you about two patients: Bob, who is 58 years old, and Joe, who is 60 years old. Bob and Joe were neighbours, and both suffered major heart attacks resulting in quadruple bypass surgeries within two weeks of each other.

Case Study 5 - Bob

Bob worked out regularly and enthusiastically every single morning despite being a senior executive working 50 to 70 hours per week. He had a serious genetic heart condition that resulted in his heart attack. During his recovery, he was able to get out of his hospital bed in record time unassisted. Anyone who has ever had a major heart operation knows that getting out of bed on your own is tremendously difficult. After a few short weeks, he recovered at home without going to cardiac rehab, as under the COVID restrictions, he was not permitted to attend recovery programs. Within a matter of weeks, he was out gardening and walking more than 5 km a day.

Case Study 6 - Joe

Across the street from him, his neighbour Joe had a rather different experience.

Although Joe did not have any genetic heart conditions, he still had a heart attack. Prior to his heart attack, he blamed his lack of time for his inability to exercise and prepare healthy meals. As he stood in his garage smoking, Joe watched in envy as his neighbour gardened, enjoyed long walks, and performed routine tasks around his house effortlessly. He blamed his inability to attend cardiac rehab as the reason for the slow recovery. Joe became depressed as he could see how quickly his neighbour recovered and returned to his normal life. Only two years his senior, Joe could barely get out of bed. Walking was certainly not a possibility for him. Unfortunately for Joe, his lack of exercise and poor diet had a serious impact on his physical and emotional recovery.

Bob took ownership of his health despite his genetic condition, not allowing it to determine his fate. Both Bob and Joe were also visited by their white swans—which you will recall is an expected event with potentially devastating consequences, but their outcomes were drastically different.

Excuses Are the Enemy of Success

If you insist on being the victim, then you become the victim. Our genes do not necessarily determine our fates. Our attitudes determine our fates.

If you have used the following excuses, then you are not alone. As a family physician, I heard all too many patients make statements like these in response to my recommendations to take action and control of their situation by implementing healthy habits.

"I don't have time to exercise."

"I can't exercise because my back hurts."

"I have no time for myself because I have kids."

" I have no time for self-care because I am too busy."

Read this quote and guess when it was written:

"Those who think they have no time for bodily exercise will sooner or later have to find time for illness." *Edward Stanley*

Answer: It was written two centuries ago. It just goes to show that the excuses of not having enough time to exercise are not a modern-day phenomenon. Furthermore, even before all the scientific data proving the importance of exercise, philosophers were already aware of its importance.

Our excuses limit our successes.

But I Just Don't Have Time

Imagine your gas tank warning light comes on, and you didn't have time to fill up. You are driving to an important meeting, and you run out of gas. It is pouring rain outside. You have to walk to the gas station five blocks away, get the gas, and carry it back to your car. You now arrive late for your meeting, walking in soaking wet with rain and smelling like gas. Not only that but during your next tune-up, your mechanic tells you that you have caused damage to your car engine because this is the third time you have done that.

How long would it have taken if you filled up your tank before it ran empty?

The same applies to our health. People who look after their health, mentally and physically, are more productive. They get more done. They are sick less often. There is so much time lost when people become ill or have to spend time on medical tests, procedures, and doctors' appointments.

Despite this, people insist that they absolutely cannot find an extra five minutes in their day. How much free time do you think you have daily? How much free time do you think research indicates people actually have?

Five and a half hours! This was shown in a study by Dr. Deborah Cohen, a senior physician-researcher, on several thousand participants around the globe. The research looked at the free time people have after time spent on work, sleep, commuting, housework, and childcare. Guess what most of that free time was spent on?

You guessed it—screen time like watching TV and scrolling social media. Social media is junk food for the mind. It is okay to indulge a little, but a lot is damaging. It is addictive and not beneficial.

What would it look like if you took half an hour of that time every day for exercise instead? And another half an hour to nourish your mind through meditation?

Do you really need to know what your old co-worker is wearing for the wedding? Or who that singer is dating?

Every time we practice doing the wrong thing, we become better at doing the wrong thing until it becomes a habit. We develop pathways in our brains that lead us to the same old patterns repeatedly.

Your path to success starts when *you* start to take responsibility to do the right thing instead of blaming others for your failures. It starts when you switch from saying, " I *can't* because..." to " I *can* because..." Once you take responsibility for your own health, you have the freedom to move forward, rather than getting stuck in the same old cycle.

We need to develop the habits for excellence as if our life depends on it because our life does depend on it. Developing habits for excellence enables us to stay ahead of the curve.

Questions to Ponder

Think of an example of good advice that you have been given by a professional to introduce a healthy habit. Now answer the following questions:

Have I taken action on those habits? If not, what reasons do I have for not implementing those new habits? Dig with an unbiased and open mind.

_____
_____
_____

Did some of the "reasons" include other people's names, perhaps? Is it possible I am blaming others for my actions?

_____
_____
_____

Are those reasons, or are they excuses? This is a tough challenge, but we have to look in the mirror in order to impact positive change and gain control.

_____
_____
_____

Action Plans

Action plan #1: Drop the excuses and blame.

"If you really want to do it, there are no excuses." Bruce Nauman

Own up to what ails you. Is it constant fatigue because you don't get enough sleep or enough exercise? Or because your dog has a healthier diet than you do? Owning the problem is the first step in moving forward and taking action to correct what needs to be corrected.

How do we motivate ourselves to take action if we just don't feel like it?

Let's say you have written down the Implementation/Intention exercise from Reflection 2. But you still tell yourself you are too tired to go for a walk or run. Or you have too many things on your mind to remember.

Action plan #2: Modify your environment.

There are two ways to modify your environment. These strategies are described in detail in James Clear's book *Atomic Habits* and proven to be effective in many research studies:

Stimulus control.

Put things in your environment to remind you of your goals. Our brains like to conserve energy and take shortcuts. Make it easier for your brain to remember what you want it to remember.

For example, put your running shoes in the hallway where you can see them easily. Or display a calendar on your fridge, where you draw a big checkmark each day you have done your exercise. This activates your brain's reward system when you see that you have followed through with your exercise intentions, which motivates you to continue.

In business, there is something called a Performance Gap, which is the difference between an intended performance and the actual performance. Think of it as a "knowing and doing gap." We know what to do; we just don't do it.

We all suffer from performance gaps in our personal lives. We know we need to exercise more and eat better, but often we do not do it. We need to close that gap. By stocking our fridge with more fruits and vegetables, we make it easier to do what we need to do.

What is the second way to modify my environment?

Get rid of temptations

Make it less visible. For example, if your problem is plopping on the couch to watch TV instead of going to exercise, move the TV to a less visible location. Or if the problem is eating junk food at night, then do not keep any junk food in the house. Willpower goes MIA when we are tired from making decisions all day. The brain wants to default to hedonism.

Action plan #3: Practice the 2-minute rule

Let's say you have put down that you will exercise by taking a thirty-minute walk every night after dinner. It is now Tuesday night, and you simply feel too exhausted. What do you do? Do just two minutes of it.

What is the point of walking for only two minutes?

By the time you put on your shoes to go outside for a walk, chances are you will not stop at two minutes. Even if you do stop after two minutes, you would still have trained your brain to develop the habit, and you are less likely to beat yourself up for not doing it. When it comes to building a habit, neuroscience shows how often you do something matters more than how long you do it.

Learn to love the process, not the goal. Be ambitious about the effort you put in daily but focus not on the result. Believe in the process.

The beauty of developing good habits is that once the habit is formed, you do not have to think about it. You just do it. When was that last time you got up in the morning and asked yourself whether you should brush your teeth?

Our brain loves that because it does not have to waste energy making decisions, freeing it up to do other things.

Reflection 4: Killing it with Kindness

*"When you have learned compassion for yourself,
compassion for others is automatic."*
~Henepola Gunaratana

Lesson from COVID-19

BC: There has been so many novel viruses in the past few decades that did not result in a global disaster. How will this particular virus manages to become a pandemic? Is it because it is more lethal or more contagious than the others?

AC: How mind-blowing it is that this simple virus without the ability to plan and strategize will succeed in bringing the world population to its knees. The genius in this virus is not how deadly it is, but how kind it is, how it will manage to infect so many people without them knowing it because the symptoms are so mild, if there are any symptoms at all. This allows a huge swath of the population to deliver the virus for free. It is incredibly efficient because it is kind to most people. It does not harm much of the people it infects.

It is our reactions versus our responses to the virus that will determine the extent of the damage incurred. New Zealand and Iceland, for example, have leaders who will demonstrate compassion and authenticity during the crisis. For these qualities, they will be praised around the world.

If you recall, Jacinda Ardern, the prime minister of New Zealand, inspired the world a year prior to the pandemic with her compassion and decisiveness in her handling of an attack in her country, which killed 49 people. The attack was from an individual who had access to weapons. She immediately responded to that situation by banning all automatic weapons. She did not hesitate, and this action is what struck a chord around the world. She didn't take weeks to decide or review with committees and debate. She immediately put this change into action. Quick, clear, decisive, and appropriate action. Her expressions and words demonstrated genuine empathy for the victims of the attack, as well as anger with the attacker. Why should this be so refreshing and unexpected?

Hatred is destructive. But anger can be different. Sometimes anger can be motivating. When anger motivates people to do the right things, hatred must be taken out of the equation. Within ten days, Prime Minister Ardern was able to ban all assault rifles and semi-automatic weapons, demonstrating that compassion does not equate with weakness.

Because of her evident compassion and empathy, people will listen when she speaks against the virus. She will be able to gain people's trust, so there will be cooperation with the mandates and policies. If you want cooperation, make the policies transparent and lead with authenticity and by example.

Contrasting this, when leaders loudly advocate and incite hatred and divisiveness, chaos and riots will ensue. Their actions will set the bar low for human behaviour. Those places will fail in controlling the pandemic because of a lack of trust and compliance.

You may recall the Aesop fable about an argument between the sun and the wind as to who is the strongest. To settle the dispute, they challenged each other to remove the coat of a traveller. The wind began blasting the traveller with all his might, but the harder he blew, the tighter the traveller gripped his coat. The wind eventually retreated from exhaustion. As the sun takes his turn, he begins to emanate a warm glow onto the traveller. The traveller relaxes and starts to unbutton his coat. As the sun's rays continue to grow warmer, the traveller eventually removed his coat.

It is not he who yells the loudest that is the most powerful. It is the soft-spoken. We can conquer the virus with kindness. To get ahead of the curve, our kindness and concern for others will result in people complying with the rules of physical distancing and mask-wearing for the sake of others. These behaviours will lead to a reduction in infection rates and confer protection to those who are vulnerable.

Why else will the infection rate spread so quickly in some countries?

One interesting thing about COVID-19 infections is that about half the people with the infection will have no symptoms, while others will have very mild symptoms. As mentioned previously, obesity is one of the major risk factors for more severe symptoms. Recall that the U.S. has one of the highest obesity rates in the world, with an obesity rate in adults of 42%. That is almost half of the population. This applies even to young people between the ages of 20 to 29, within which 40% of people are obese.

How will that translate to their infection rate? The U.S. will have one of the worst infections and death rates in the world. There are many reasons for that. Once the dust settles, it will be beneficial and significant for our global health and wellbeing to see how much of that can be attributed to their high obesity rates.

However, it is important not to stigmatize obesity. There is already an epidemic of fat-shaming in North America. This current fact of obesity being a risk factor for more severe infections should not be a catalyst for blaming people who struggle with weight control and implying they are inflicting harm to themselves mentally or physically. It cannot be viewed as a character flaw because there are so many nuances related to it, both on a personal and societal level. Compassion and kindness need to be applied to affect change. This includes people applying self-compassion to themselves.

What we learn from being compassionate during COVID-19

Compassion is an essential attribute for an effective leader. It fosters trust and trust, in turn, fosters loyalty and cooperation. These attitudes help organizations stay ahead of the curve.

"But what's in it for me," you ask? "Don't good guys finish last?" As it turns out, science shows otherwise.

Cultivating compassion also benefits the person practicing the attribute. Studies indicate that when people show compassion toward others, they benefit themselves by becoming more at peace with themselves, which increases their happiness. Mindfulness training is amazingly effective in increasing one's ability to develop compassion. It is also effective in helping us develop self-awareness, so we can respond calmly and rationally to stressful situations, rather than reacting and lashing out.

Nourish with Self Compassion

Here is an unfamiliar fact that can be exceedingly difficult to stomach. The virus will not only kill through infections. It will also kill indirectly because of people's reactions.

Dr. Roger McIntyre, a Toronto psychiatrist and university professor, will estimate that the suicide rate from unemployment alone because of lockdown measures will increase by 27% per year. That translates to the lives of 4,000 more people in Canada. This is equivalent to the number of people needed to fill twenty movie theatres. This is not due to the virus. This is due to our reactions.

Death is the ultimate cost of lack of self-compassion. It is an extremely high price to pay.

To cultivate self-compassion, think about this question for a moment. Which of these voices do you find more motivating?

"I can't believe you missed your exercise again today! No wonder why you can never reach your goals. You can't even get your ass out of bed to exercise." This is the voice of the antagonist.

Or the voice of the gentle, empathetic friend?

"Yes, so you missed your exercise today because you just feel you cannot squeeze in the time. How about getting in that walk tomorrow before checking your Facebook to ensure you have enough time?"

Self-compassion is bringing kindness to your own suffering. Not only does it increase your resilience and well-being, but it also increases your success in achieving health-related goals such as weight loss, exercise, and smoking cessation. When you stop beating yourself up, you are more motivated and energized. People with self-compassion are not afraid of failure, and this makes them more resourceful and creative. They are more willing to get back to the drawing board and try again. Self-compassion is motivating. For a lot of people, feeling self-compassion is difficult. If that is your case, you can bring on self-compassion by talking to yourself as you would your five-year-old self or someone you care about.

You may be wondering whether self-compassion is the same as selfishness. Well, unlike selfishness, self-compassion is about kindness rather than self-centeredness. When you can show compassion to yourself, you increase your personal resources, which will give you the fuel to offer compassion to others. When your emotional gas tank is empty, it is difficult to offer compassion to others.

Those that run on an empty compassion tank run the risk of compassion fatigue, which is an extremely destructive state. It is often seen in caring professions like physicians, nurses, and teachers. This is why these professionals have such high levels of burnout-- they have nothing left in their emotional gas tank to give to others. Fill up your gas tank.

Questions to Ponder:

How do I look after my closest loved ones, perhaps a child or a spouse?

_____

_____

_____

How do I look after myself?

_____

_____

_____

Once you value yourself, you will look after yourself the same way you look after a prized possession.

- Do you feed that body with good nutritious food, rather than mindlessly shoving in processed foods full of damaging chemicals?
- Do you allow the body to exercise so that the muscles remain powerful and flexible, and the bones remain strong?
- Do you nourish the mind with positive thoughts, read information from credible sources rather than looking at sensation headlines, and taking things at face value?

Action Plans

Practice self- compassion.

Kristin Neff, one of the most prolific researchers on self-compassion, describes these steps whenever you feel stressed or upset.

1. First, pause and acknowledge it. Place the palm of your right hand over your heart. This activates your parasympathetic nervous system, which tells your body to slow down the heart rate and decrease blood pressure. It calms you down. Often, we are in such automatic pilot mode that we are not even aware that we are angry, anxious, or sad. Then we lash out at the people we love without realizing why. Having awareness is the first step to responding rationally.
2. Second, you show yourself kindness. If you find it difficult to feel self-compassion, you can try talking to yourself the same way you would talk to a loved one or picture how you would talk to yourself if you were your five-year-old self.
3. Third, recognize the common humanity. Tell yourself, "Yes, I am feeling upset. This is normal because suffering is part of life. I accept myself as I am."

Just think, would you ever say to a five-year-old child, " I don't like you because you are _____(fill in the blank with whatever awful thing it is you tell yourself)" Why is it that we would say these comments to ourselves?

Just like any skill, the more often you do this, the better you become at it.

Regular meditation practice is a powerful tool to help increase your compassion, both to yourself and others

.

Reflection 5: Some of Us Are in This Together

"Remember, there is no such thing as a small act of kindness. Every act creates a ripple with no logical end."
~Scott Adams

Lesson from COVID-19

> BC: How do the cultural differences amongst countries influence their responses to the pandemic and what impact does culture have?

AC: Countries whose cultures are based on collectivism like Japan, Hong Kong, and Singapore will stay ahead of the curve during the pandemic. These are countries whose people's actions are based on the premise that their actions affect others as a whole. Their cultures are made up of individuals that consider the needs of the community over that of the individual, and group cohesion is highly valued. They have the "We are all in this together, so lets all cooperate so we can all benefit" mentality. These countries will do well in bringing down the infection outbreaks quickly. More locally in provinces across Canada, including my home province of Ontario, it will be quite heartwarming to see that we will have a huge number of nurses and doctors volunteering to come out of their retirement to help during the pandemic if the system becomes overwhelmed. There will be numerous anecdotes of people stepping up to do more frontline work to

BC: What about countries whose cultures are based on individualism like the U.S. and U.K, which is more about individual's "rights"?

AC: As a broad generalization, countries based on individualism exists in a culture of "everyone for themselves." It is not a simple black and white scenario, as there are advantages to individualism. However, there is a tendency toward less cohesiveness in their relationships. In some of these places, there will be a shift from the attitude of altruism to selfish acts. There will be news reports of violence toward store clerks as a result of mask refusal because wearing masks is seen as an infringement on individual rights. The price they will pay is rampant infection rates and chaos. People attacking each other, with behaviours reminiscent of *Lord of the Flies*, except these are adults. There will be a great deal of xenophobia. The mentality becomes "me" versus "them." This phenomenon is clear in the graph below from Johns Hopkins University based on data from April 2020. I expect the graph will be even more divergent if data from later months of the pandemic were used.

COVID-19 infections rates vs a measure of societal collectivism / individualism
Total infections to date per million people

Dev. Asia/China
GPS tracking; credit card receipt logs; close circuit television monitoring; mandatory quarantine, electronic wristbands and saliva testing of incoming travelers; mandatory smartphone "virus passport" apps

cluster significance coefficient 82%

Source: Johns Hopkins University, IMF, G. Hofstede Cultural Dimensions (2015), JPMAM. Diamonds represent cluster centroids. April 17, 2020

Having scientific knowledge and resources mean nothing if you don't have the leadership that can inspire the cooperation of the public.

Okay, enough depressing stuff. Now for something uplifting. Studies from children to adults show that humans are innately kind and altruistic. Studies comparing different cultures and animal species also show that groups with more kindness and altruism are more successful. Humans are innately good. What's more, that goodness can be trained.

Altruism and collectivism are stronger than selfishness. As a society, altruism and kindness promote social connections, which is important for our wellbeing and cooperation. As a result, society becomes stronger.

Here is a fun fact. Did you know social science showed that people who demonstrate kindness are considered more attractive?

> BC: Hmmm. That means people can save a fortune on Botox injections by practicing kindness instead.

How altruism can help us stay ahead of the curve in our personal wellbeing

My friend Calvin has three adorable sons and a wife with a heart of gold. Calvin is one of the kindest, most compassionate doctors you could meet. Over the Christmas holidays, his lovely wife Barb spent hours at home cutting the thorns off rose stems to ensure there were no sharp points. The next day, with the roses in a beautiful basket prepared by Barb, Calvin would bring his sons to visit his patients in the hospital--patients who were not able to go home during the holidays. His sons went around the ward to each patient, handing out roses personally.

I am smiling just thinking about it. Such a simple gesture, but I am certain that it left a smile on every patient's face for a long time. Not only that, but I have no doubt his sons also learned a valuable lesson on the joys of kindness. It is safe to say that Calvin's altruistic acts have benefitted not only patients he gave the roses to but also their families when they learn of such thoughtfulness shown to their loved ones, and his sons in learning about compassion. These good feelings help everyone stay ahead of the curve.

When patients ask if I get the flu shot annually, I tell them yes, but not just for myself. Mostly, it was so that I do not pass the flu to my patients. It is not only about our freedom. It is about consideration for others.

Kindness is also contagious. In a team setting and in our social groups, it increases the collective cohesiveness and cooperation. When we are negative and stressed out, our mood affects three degrees of our social connections. Happiness also spreads by three degrees. Let's say you are happy. So, you treat your co-worker Jane with kindness and support. Jane goes home in a good mood and treats her husband, George, with more kindness. Her husband, George, visits his parents and spread the happy feelings to them. Just by being happier yourself, you can potentially increase the happiness level of your co-worker, her husband, *and* his parents. You can see how something as simple as being kind and positive at work can make such an impact as it is passed along like a positive virus. Even if you do not care enough about yourself to become calmer, healthier, and have more patience, do it for people you care about by adopting practices that will allow you to become a better person.

We can all do with a cultural shift to courtesy and protecting others, cultivating concern for others' happiness and wellbeing. When we achieve this, we will also benefit ourselves.

If altruism is about helping other people, how does it benefit us? WIIFM (What's in it for me)?

When people are depressed, their focus turns inwards. Their narrative becomes only about themselves. Me, me, me. They carry on with feeling only sorry for themselves:

"Poor me, I can never get a break."

"My life is so unfair."

"Nobody cares about me."

They can only see their own pain and suffering. But when people decide to help others, their focus shifts outwards to other people. They begin to see that they are not the only ones that suffer. They begin to understand that suffering is part of common humanity. Wanting to help others gives them a sense of purpose, which increases their resilience. Resilience needs a sense of purpose to grow. It also energizes people and increases their sense of contentment. People who volunteer, for example, are in better physical health, have more social connections, and live longer. Social connection is vital to wellbeing. So helping others is actually good for our wellbeing and helps us stay ahead of the curve.

Question to Ponder

How can I be of service to others? (This may include not just people in your inner circle but also in the community at large, like volunteering at a senior center)

_____

_____

_____

_____

Action Plan

This is an exercise on kindness from the University of California Berkeley.

Perform five random acts of kindness for one day each week. Do this for six weeks.

Try to make the acts different. They can be small acts, like checking in on a friend by phone, or getting coffee for a co-worker, or helping pick up groceries for a neighbour who has difficulties getting out.

Record these acts to help you remember them.

Random Acts of Kindness

Week 1

_____
_____
_____

Week 2

_____
_____
_____

Week 3

_____
_____
_____

Week 4

_____

_____

_____

Week 5

_____

_____

_____

Week 6

_____

_____

_____

This exercise has been found to increase people's happiness levels. Even more than that, kindness has a ripple effect.

Reflection 6: Hazards of Infodemic and the Dark Side of Hope

"It is easier to fool someone than it is to convince them that they have been fooled." ~Mark Twain

Lesson from COVID-19

AC: Which of these two headlines will grab your attention more? Scientists show the COVID-19 will live on surfaces for days! Or science shows the COVID-19 on surfaces are unlikely to cause infections.

BC: The first one of course.

AC: Exactly. The first headline will drive fear, so people will remember it. Besides COVID-19, there is another illusive pandemic spreading covertly without most people noticing. This is the trend of infodemics.

> BC: What is infodemic?

> AC: Infodemic refers to an excess of information, both true and false. The pandemic will really amplify how many deceptions are placed upon unsuspecting people. Infodemic is more insidious than fake news, making it more difficult to detect. There will be deceptions about the number of people affected by the virus, the number of deaths, dubious cures, and false hopes about how quickly a vaccine will be ready. Even professionals like doctors and scientists will, at times, be deceived by preprints of studies promising cures before the studies are properly peer-reviewed.

This is the Kruger-Dunning effect I referred to earlier. Often, the less one knows, the more they think they know. People think they know enough, but they don't know enough to know when they are wrong. This applies to everyone, including doctors and university professors.

How does misinformation spread? Often a lot of misinformation comes from social media. Frightening stories that are posted may or may not be true, and even if true, may be rare. Emotion is what drives people to read these stories and spread them. Emotional stories, especially frightening ones, have a much greater impact on our brains than rational scientific ones, so we remember them better. We ignore or forget the rational, calm news. The misinformation will spread like wildfire. It is difficult to control once it starts. Good journalism has contributed tremendously to our knowledge of numerous important issues. However, some journalists follow the motto, "If it bleeds, it leads." Because calm news does not attract attention, there is less of it. Next thing you know, there is massive collective hysteria.

Let me explain why the first headline is misleading, even though it is not false.

Infodemic Trap #1: Fear

When sensational headlines drive panic, they overwhelm people's rational brains, or the executive brain I mentioned in Reflection 2. Even if the information is correct, there are misinterpretations of the information when people do not have the background knowledge to understand them. We cannot be experts in everything, so this applies even to people with science backgrounds.

The media throws in scientific terms and data; people read them and think they understand, then they interpret the data based on their biases and fears. To add fuel to the fire, most people have difficulty truly understanding risk just by looking at numbers because the numbers are not given in any context.

Early in the pandemic, there will be a great deal of headlines like the one above talking about how long the virus can survive on various surfaces. It all sounds quite credible because the studies come from legitimate sources. So, people start wearing gloves and wiping down everything they buy. People will become fearful of touching anything on store shelves. Public bathrooms will be shut down because of the fear of contaminated surfaces. Businesses will be disinfecting chairs and tables to the point that they are more sterile than standards set in hospital operating rooms for open heart surgeries.

These "preventative" measures are as useful as wearing a tinfoil hat to prevent diabetes. Here is a little-known fact. Those studies will be based on artificial conditions. According to one of the most respected medical journals, *The Lancet*,[1] the dose of virus used in these studies is equivalent to, wait for this...10,000-100,000 infected people in one small area. That is equal to the total number of people attending five NHL games! The public simply is not aware of this because either: the journalists reporting this news are unaware themselves because they don't have the analytical background or time to interpret the minutiae of scientific data, or they choose not to report this crucial aspect because fear sells. What many people do not know is that you

---

[1] Exaggerated risk of transmission of COVID-19 by fomites. *The Lancet*

need a certain dose of the virus before you can get infected, and you cannot pick up this dose from touching surfaces in the community.

Did you know that apple seeds contain cyanide? And that if you eat 100-500 apple seeds, it is possible to suffer acute cyanide poisoning? Should we start banning apples from all children in case they swallow a seed?

Here is the bigger problem: the WHO (World Health Organization) *and* CDC (Center for Disease Control) will announce in July that the risk of transmission from contaminated surfaces is negligible; unfortunately, this message will be drowned out by a multitude of fear-inducing headlines. Despite this evidence, policies about frantically sterilizing every single surface will not be changed to reflect the new knowledge. Many resources will be put into these utterly useless, expensive, and ineffectual "preventative measures." Surely there are healthier and more productive things we can do with our time.

Infodemic Trap #2: The Dark Side of Hope

> BC: What about information giving people hope? Isn't that helpful?

> AC: Hope, for the most part, is good. It's motivating. It's the energy that keeps people moving forward. Hope prevents the death of despair. But one of the laws of the universe is Yin and Yang. Where there is good, there is also bad. Hope also has a dark side.

What is its dark side? Hope is wanting. The object of our wanting is not always within our control. We want the pandemic to disappear. We want to see our friends and families in person again rather than on a screen. We want the economy to stop bleeding. These wants can lead to suffering. Wanting is a hunger. Sometimes people deceive themselves because they need hope. This can lead to false hope.

Infodemic can also lead to false hope. Every time a headline screams out about a promising vaccine here, another promising vaccine there, people think its availability is just around the corner. They are not aware that these vaccines are still many months away before they can be proven safe and effective, and many more months before they can be given to the general population. Or they believe the myriad of advertised natural concoctions that will protect them from becoming infected. False hope leads to delusions. Notice how so many hockey parents believe their children are the next Sidney Crosby or Hayley Wickenheiser until they discover they are not?

False hopes make people irrational. There will be people getting sick from taking unproven cures. During the mass hysteria at the start of the pandemic, many people will listen to all sorts of pseudoscience advice and end up harming themselves by bathing with bleach or taking unproven treatments that result in grave injuries to themselves, even death.

Today's society is full of information but lacking in wisdom.

Infodemic Trap #3: Deception by Information

"When you mix politics with science, you get politics." ~John Barry

What do you think he was referring to? This quote was taken from John Barry's book on the 1918 influenza pandemic entitled "The Great Influenza." It will aptly describe the Pandemic of 2020. History indeed repeats itself. We must heed to science, even if science continues to evolve. Science should be non-partisan. We need to learn from history and heed its mistakes.

Deception can also be achieved by manipulating information. A glaring case of this is cutting funding to testing sites in the U.S. by the federal government because more testing will show more people infected. By not having the data on the number of people infected, they can deceive the public of the infection rates. This is akin to my patient declining screening for his colon cancer despite being in the high-risk group so that he can feel better about not finding out he has cancer. Research will show that increased testing early in the pandemic allows more data for scientists to work with to bring the infection under control, just like how cancer screening in high-risk groups allows early cancer detection and increases the chance of cure rather than death. We need policies that are data-driven, not emotion, or politically driven.

How Infodemic Programs our Bodies

Do you realize that you are programming your mind each time you read sensational headlines without critical thinking? Many people will be getting stressed out listening to negative and frightening news all day, looking at numbers they don't know how to effectively interpret. You have no doubt heard the saying, "You are what you eat." What's more relevant during the pandemic is, "You are what you think."

Surround ourselves with negative thoughts, and we become negative. Surround ourselves with hate, and we become hateful. Surround ourselves with frightening news all day, we become frightened. Eventually, we end up with a personality so noxious that it can be used as a human repellent.

Our body then becomes accustomed to being in a frightened state all the time. We end up conditioning our body to be in a constant anxious mode or program our thinking with negativity. Eventually, we suffer panic attacks even in the absence of anything dangerous because we have trained our bodies this way.

But here's the good news. As much as we can program our bodies into this fretful state, we can also program them into a positive state through exercise, mindfulness training, and connecting with positive people. We can also avoid the trap of infodemic by stopping clicking on sensational headlines, limiting the quantity of the information we take in, and sticking to credible sources. We need to develop humility and recognize that we cannot all be experts when trying to interpret data that is presented.

As one of the first nations that will declare itself virus-free on June 8, New Zealand Prime Minister Ardern will deliver this simple message: "We almost certainly will see cases again. It is a reality of this virus. If and when it occurs, we have to make sure we are prepared."

There is no fear-mongering, no giving false hope. Ardern's message will mix optimism with preparedness. It is this transparency that will allow her nation to stay ahead of the curve.

Understanding that infodemics leads to deceptions and false hopes can help us stay ahead of the curve

Case Study 7 - Richard

Richard is an intelligent, large man with a robust voice. He held a high-ranking job, with many people reporting to him. He commanded the confidence of someone who is deeply knowledgeable when he speaks. He worked hard at his job and was now enjoying a well-deserved retirement. He spends his spare time reading and watching TV.

Richard, speaking excitedly: "Hi Doc, guess what, I'm taking a teaspoon of cinnamon every day for my diabetes."

Me: "Okay...But your diabetes bloodwork results are still getting worse. Are you physically exercising?"

Richard: "No."

Me: "Your weight has gone up since your last visit. Are you still eating the bacon and eggs breakfast every morning?"

Richard: "Yes. Every morning at my favourite diner. I am not giving that up."

Me: "I've already prescribed the maximum doses on all your diabetes medications. How are you going to get it under control?"

Richard perks up brightly: "That's why I'm taking the cinnamon. I brought you this newspaper article that says cinnamon helps lower blood sugar."

Me: "Yes, but by how much? Your blood sugar needs to improve by at least 50%. The cinnamon only helps lower it by a minuscule amount, not even enough to reflect on your bloodwork."

Richard looks down sullenly, "It's a lot easier taking the cinnamon than doing the things you are suggesting!"

Despite his high IQ, Richard focused on what he felt was the silver bullet of having a teaspoon of cinnamon. He was attached to his long-standing style of eating and remaining sedentary, so he deluded himself that he would not need to heed any of the proven behavioural changes which are far more effective. Now let's turn to Kim, who followed a different approach.

Case Study 8 - Kim

Kim is a fifty-eight-year-old professional well-loved by everyone at her work because of her dedication and compassion. She carries with her a radiant smile everywhere she goes. Her positivity is infectious. Her generosity touched many people who crossed her path. Kim's biggest struggle was her morbid obesity. Even though she was aware of the importance of exercise and diet, she always had time for everyone else except herself.

Over the course of several months, Kim's right knee had progressively become so painful that by the time she came to see me, she could not walk from the parking lot to my examination room. I had to see her at the front of the clinic closest to the parking lot. X-rays indicated a completely worn out knee joint because of excess weight over the years. Based on the x-rays, Kim would require a knee replacement.

It would take over a year before Kim could get an appointment to see an orthopedic surgeon and another year of being on the waiting list before she can get the surgery. I advised Kim that the surgeon would not agree to the surgery until she lost at least fifty pounds because excess weight reduces the chance of successful outcomes and increases complications from the surgery.

Kim was determined. "Doc, just tell me what I need to do. I'm going to do it."

Because Kim was unable to walk, I suggested she start with a stationary bike and cycle regularly. Kim committed to that with the vigour of a golden retriever wagging her tail upon seeing her owner return home. She started with five minutes on her bike twice daily because her legs could only tolerate that amount. Eventually, she built up to a total of one hour of cycling daily. She attended regular physiotherapy sessions to assist with her mobility. Kim was also dedicated to eating healthy meals.

Here's the knockout punch. By the time Kim arrived at her appointment with the orthopedic surgeon, she had not only lost eighty pounds but was also able to walk for miles without any difficulty. Because she was so functionally capable, despite her x-ray results, the surgeon advised Kim she no longer required surgery.

Really basic stuff, right? Kim did not research any magical diets or buy into any of the miracle machines that promise to vibrate your body into the size of a supermodel. She achieved the results through perseverance and simple proven rudimentary practices.

Numerous studies indicate that lifestyle behaviours, like exercise and healthy eating, are far more effective than medications for preventing and treating diabetes, along with many other medical conditions. Instead of focusing their energy on the proven strategies, many people look to quick fixes. This is why there are so many scams selling dubious cures. What is the cost of these misguided remedies? At the minimum, there is a cost of money and time wasted; at its worst, harm to the body, including death.

This has occurred all the time throughout human history, not just during the pandemic. Our current information world allows false claims to spread all the more quickly and effectively than before.

There are many promotions of products making preposterous claims like "Shed fifty pounds without exercise!", "Develop muscles of an Olympian God!" or "Look twenty years younger!" Whatever your heart desires, there is a product for it. Purveyors of these products exploit people's wants and attachments to ideas of looking a certain way: prettier, younger, more hair (only on top of the head, not the body). We fall prey to these false claims because of our attachments.

Infodemic Traps Our Wants

Things we are attached to can often be outside of our control. This can be our attachment to not just our ideas but also our possessions, our status, looks, or our youth. Attachment is a *want*. When we do not get what we want, we suffer. To experience contentment in life, we need to let go of our attachments and wants. Attachments trap, while detachments free us.

Because of our wants, we can develop false hope. So, we often delude ourselves.

You are now thinking: "Not me. I don't delude myself. I'm too smart for that."

Intelligence does not protect us from delusions. We use information to justify our delusions. We interpret the information to align with our beliefs. Recognize that it is extremely easy to fool ourselves. We all do that because of our cognitive biases. We need to accept when we are wrong. Only then can we learn.

Expand Your Mind

If we insist on seeing the world through a keyhole, then our world will be the size of a keyhole. If we spend much of our time reading or watching questionable or negative news, then our world will be a dangerous, evil place we watch daily. We can also delude ourselves when we take in a junk food diet of information from unreliable sources. We will then connect with a tribe who thinks the same unconstructive beliefs, making our world a smaller place.

Here is a metaphor relating to that idea. In ancient China, women's feet were bound tightly to prevent them from growing, as small feet were considered beautiful. But the feet become deformed, rendering their owner unable to walk properly or run.

If you bind your mind through questionable information and not allow it to grow, then your mind too will be rendered small and disabled, not allowing you to see the truth around you.

Let go of your attachments to your wants, so your mind can be free and open to seeing reality. When you become aware of how infodemic can influence your perceptions, you can liberate yourself from it and stay ahead of the curve.

Questions to Ponder

What material am I choosing to listen to or read?

Begin keeping a diary tracking the data of frequency and nature of intake. For example, write down how much of your information comes from Facebook. Track the time you spend on Facebook and your phone.

How is it helping me grow as a human being? How is it contributing to my knowledge?

_____

_____

_____

What kind of people (*thinkers*) do I listen to? Do they keep me in a tiny prison of small-minded thinking, or do they expand my views of the universe?

_____

_____

_____

Do I just want to be right, or do I want to know the truth? Ask yourself this every time you encounter credible information that contradicts your beliefs. This requires humility. Play devil's advocate by having a healthy debate taking an opposing side with an open mind.

Action Plan

> "All are lunatics, but he who can analyze his delusion is called a philosopher." ~Ambrose Bierce

In Malcolm Gladwell's book Blink, he discusses how we make split-second decisions based on our experiences and assumptions. Constantly ask yourself if your thoughts are accurate.

- Ask yourself what your perceptions are. Recognize the possibility that your perceptions may not be a reality. Reality does not care what you think. Reality is reality.
- Recognize how your own perceptions can be distorted by virtue of your past experience, your hopes, and the people around you.
- Respect others' perceptions because there is a possibility they are right.
- Be willing to admit you may be wrong if credible evidence suggests it. This takes courage. Having the flexibility to change your opinion is more powerful than rigidity.
- Do not get too attached to your perceptions and ideas.

Reflection 7: I Can't Believe Me

"I would never die for my beliefs because I might be wrong."
~Bertrand Russel

Lesson from COVID-19

> AC: Pssssst. Want to hear a secret? Science is the truth, but it is not the ultimate truth. The truth changes. Thus, science at times is more about probabilities.
>
> There will be this huge debate on masks during the pandemic. Initially in Canada, wearing masks will be considered ineffective. However, new data will suggest that if most people wear masks, even though there is little benefit in protecting themselves, the benefit lies in protecting others if the mask wearer is infectious. That turns wearing masks into an altruistic act, not as an encroachment on one's freedom of choice.

> BC: So, the facts changed. Isn't science supposed to be absolute?

AC: Most things are not absolute. Information of "facts" will evolve rapidly, with scientists from all over the world dedicating their work and collecting data on effective ways to control the pandemic. What is considered a scientific fact may change based on new evidence. Often, scientists will make statements but add that they may change their assertions within days as new information surfaces.

Scientists constantly question themselves as to whether their beliefs are facts, challenging their viewpoints as they continue their search for truth. They must be willing to have the flexibility and openness to admit when they are wrong, rather than sticking with dogmatism and inflexibility which will be seen in some leaders and organizations. They remain humble. It takes much more courage to admit one is wrong, than to insist on one's wrong beliefs in the face of contrary evidence.

BC: Surely political leaders will be making mistakes also. Do they concede when this happens?

> AC: The prime minister of Norway, Erna Solberg, will be quoted at the end of May admitting that her shutdown of schools was based on fear, and she will state that even with a second wave, she will not close schools. She will recognize that her previous beliefs were wrong and will own up to it. The erroneous initial beliefs will have mistakenly driven the behaviour of shutting down schools. New evidence which will evolve shows doing that will cause more harm than good. Solberg will admit and denounce the error in thinking. That takes courage but is also a sign of great leadership. Thanks to that leadership, Norway will be one of the countries that fares well during the pandemic because she has the trust and respect of the citizens. This leads to compliance and cooperation with the mandates among the people.

Much of the policies around the world will be based on fear, not science. Given that little will be known during the early months, the extreme measures will be understandable. However, what is not excusable is when policymakers fail to change the harmful directives, and continue with measures based on fear, theatrics, or ego. Either the false beliefs are not being recognized or not acknowledged.

Policies must be based on rationality and scientific evidence rather than emotions. When leaders can recognize the errors in their directives and change course based on evolving scientific evidence, they will be able to help their people stay ahead of the curve.

Acknowledging our false beliefs and our irrationality will help us stay ahead of the curve

There is an old fable about a highly educated professor and a Zen master. People from all over the world come to seek counsel and wisdom from this Zen master.

When the scholarly professor finally arrived at the home of the Zen master, he explained how he had travelled many miles and trekked up the rugged mountain terrain on foot to arrive there. He explained how many university degrees he had and his numerous academic publications. He asked the Zen master to open his mind to enlightenment.

The Zen master invited him into his home for tea. As the Zen master poured the tea, the teacup filled. The Zen master continued pouring even when the teacup overflowed. Tea now has spilled over onto the table and onto the professor's lap.

The professor jumped back and asked why he continued to pour despite the teacup overflowing.

With a smile, the Zen master replied in a kindly manner, "Just as this teacup is full, so is your mind, full of your own ideas and opinions so that nothing can be added. Come back when it is empty."

What this fable tells us is that when you think you know everything, you will not have the capacity to take on more knowledge. When you become entrenched in your beliefs, your mind will not be able to absorb new information even in the face of data that refutes those beliefs.

> *"Knowledge is learning something every day. Wisdom is letting something go every day."* ~Zen Proverb

Human Beings Are Irrational

If you knew how ridiculously faulty our perceptions are, you would be shocked at how humans ever managed to come as far as a species as we have. If you don't believe me, just look at how many people in April will panic when their stockpile of toilet papers dipped down to fifty rolls. Here's an insider view of how our brain is so wacky. Daniel Kahneman, who won the Nobel prize for his research on cognitive biases, talks about how irrational the human mind is.

The Trap of Irrational Thinking #1: Impact Bias

Imagine you just won the lottery jackpot. Imagine all the wonderful things you can do with the money. Are you picturing how you and your family can live happily ever after? Spending the winter months on your 100-foot yacht on the Mediterranean blue seas, sipping wine, and watching the sunset? How long do you think this happiness will last? Five years? Ten? For the rest of your life?

Answer: A few months. Not even a year!

This is called impact bias: our tendency to overestimate our emotions to outcomes of events, whether it is good or bad. People who lose their jobs during the pandemic, for example, will imagine that they will never recover from their devastation. They believe their life is over. They fall into the depression of despair. People see adversity as far worse than it actually is. They ruminate on these thoughts of doom, and they behave according to these thoughts.

The Trap of Irrational Thinking #2: Availability Bias

Pop quiz. What is more contagious, COVID-19, or measles?

When we see the news reports of the daily death counts, we take the mental shortcuts that COVID-19 is a tremendously deadly and contagious virus. This is despite evidence that measles, for example, is multiple times more contagious. I have never seen patients line up to ensure their measles vaccine is up to date.

In availability heuristic, as in the above example, we are biased to think of information that first comes into our minds when evaluating an idea. Because of this flaw in thinking, we end up with people fearing Armageddon each time they leave their homes for fear of catching COVID-19 since all they have heard daily for months is the daily infection rates.

The Trap of Irrational Thinking #3: Confirmation Bias

Another type of irrational thinking is confirmation bias. Here, we listen or read only information that confirms our beliefs and ignores information that contradicts these beliefs regardless of how credible they are. People who believe that COVID-19 is extremely dangerous and hold their breath when walking past someone momentarily on the sidewalk, or won't touch any surfaces at all for fear of picking up one virus particle, will ignore reassurances from scientists that there are extremely low probabilities of catching the infection in those situations. They will only pay attention to the headlines of the daily infection rates. Without a context of what the rates mean, they cannot interpret its implications. All they see are the terrifying dangers lurking around every corner.

The Cost of False Beliefs

What do you think is more harmful, the physical or the mental traumas of the pandemic?

Studies on previous pandemics showed that people recovered faster from the physical traumas of pandemics than the mental traumas. Which means it is our *thinking* rather than the virus that resulted in more harm.

We pay for these chronic anxieties with our mental and physical wellbeing. They will drive behaviours that are harmful, stemming from our desire to gain some sense of control. These behaviours can be in the form of ingesting enough potato chips, alcohol, and drugs that would put a freshman party to shame—or spraying enough disinfectants to knock over the family Chihuahua from its fumes. Despair can lead to despondency, causing us to sit on the couch binge-watching TV until our bodies are covered with mold.

How can we combat our biases? We need to recognize the flaws in our thinking and to constantly challenge our beliefs, especially if there is compelling data showing otherwise. Our belief that we are rational thinkers is false. We need to non-identify with our perspectives and be open when the evidence violates those perspectives. This requires letting go of our ego and admitting that another perspective is correct when valid evidence is presented. In this way, we grow as human beings. We learn.

To do this, we need a genuinely curious and open mindset, the beginner's mind.

Our Beliefs Drive Our Behaviour

Next time you are lamenting on how your life sucks, think of Helen Keller. Despite being blind, deaf, and mute, she graduated from Harvard with honours. She famously said: "The only thing worse than being blind is having sight, but no vision."

You will live your present based on your vision about your future. If you envision yourself as happy, healthy, being able to be independent, travel, do whatever you wish, then you will look after your body and your mind to fulfill that vision. This is an example of intrinsic motivation. Use that vision to inspire your beliefs, so you can become the best version of yourself.

I have a confession. Sometimes it is difficult to maintain a bold vision when you fail to see results day after day. Whenever I feel discouraged, I remind myself of this story about a stonecutter.

Every day, passersby would see the stonecutter hammering away at an enormous boulder. They would ask what he is doing. "I'm trying to split this boulder into smaller pieces so they can be moved."

Day after day, under the blazing sun, the pelting rain, the stonecutter hammered away at the boulder relentlessly. Passersby would see that despite his untiring hammering, the boulder remains the same.

Until one day, as the stonecutter delivered that final hit with the hammer, the boulder split into two.

Despite our persistent efforts, it can be discouraging to not see any results and be tempted to give up and revert to old habits that do not require work. But sometimes progress is happening under the surface without our awareness. If we persevere, we will see the rewards.

Our behaviours are based on our beliefs. When we believe we can, we will. When we believe we can't, we won't. Have you ever heard yourself say these things?

"I can't lose weight because I've tried before, and I have never been successful."

" I can't exercise because I'm clumsy, and I'm embarrassed people will judge me."

"I will never get that promotion because I'm not smart enough."

Whether it is exercise, mindfulness practice, or losing weight, you may not see the results immediately. Until one day, you realize you can run up those steps with agility, fit into those pants with ease, or respond to a hostile co-worker with the calmness of a lake on a breezeless day instead of reacting with anger. Next thing you know, you become this awesome human being you aspired to be. *This* is the marvel of the right beliefs and consistent effort.

To change our behaviours, we need to change our beliefs. Cultivate beliefs that serve you well rather than hold you back. Recognizing the flaws and biases in our perceptions and being willing to change the course will help us stay ahead of the curve.

Questions to Ponder

What beliefs am I holding onto that is holding me back from enjoying my life? (Is it my negative beliefs about my abilities? Is it my beliefs about what others think of me?)

_____
_____
_____

What beliefs do I have that imprison rather than free me? (Example: Is it my idea of what a perfect parent should be? What a perfect job is? How much money I need to make?)

_____
_____
_____

How would I feel if I were to drop some of these beliefs that do not serve me well?

_____
_____
_____

Action Plans

Instead of focusing on things you cannot do, see if you can focus on what you *can* do. When you can change your beliefs, you can change your behaviour.

Look at your self-imposed roadblocks. Critically challenge your "I can't" items. Are they true impossibilities, or are they excuses to avoid the intense effort behind taking steps that result in positive and lasting change? Call yourself out on these self-imposed roadblocks, both real and imagined.

- My self-imposed roadblocks.
- Things I *can* do daily to become more content.
- Actions I need to take to do to become more content.
- When I will take those actions.

Reflection 8: Collateral Damage and Safetyism

"People at war with themselves will always cause collateral damage in the lives of those around them." ~John Mark Green

Lesson from COVID-19

> BC: Wow. The thoughts of being locked down at home for months is quite daunting, and that's knowing I'll have family that I love with me. I imagine it would be incredibly challenging for some people, especially those who are currently struggling mentally.

AC: In 2019, according to the Commonwealth Fund, the U.S. ranked last out of 11 developed countries in healthcare despite being one of the highest spenders. Canada ranked in the bottom third. This is a lower ranking than many of the European countries that spend less percentage of their GDP on healthcare. That data reflects a lack of efficiency in delivery. Which means pouring more money into the system is not the answer.

Because of inefficiencies in the healthcare system, there is no wiggle room when disaster strikes. Therefore, hospitals will have to shut down all elective medical care during the pandemic. The cost of the inefficiencies will result in collateral damage because patients whose medical care will be delayed will suffer grim consequences.

BC: What kind of consequences?

AC: Our former Ontario Medical Association president Dr. Sohail Gandhi will describe his personal examples of collateral damage from his medical practice in June in this excerpt from his article:

1. *A patient with significant stomach pain who had scans delayed for a month, only to discover cancer.*
2. *A patient who I diagnosed with melanoma, who still hasn't gotten the required wide excision, and lymph node biopsy eight weeks later.*

3. *A patient who sent me an email clearly indicating the desire to commit suicide because of the mental health effects of this pandemic (I got a hold of them, and appropriate measures have been taken).*
4. *A patient with a cough since January who still hasn't seen a specialist.*
5. *A sharp increase in patients requesting counselling or medications for the stress and depression directly caused by the effects of the pandemic.*
6. *At least five patients who were already waiting for joint replacement surgery now delayed even more. Keep in mind that I am just one comprehensive care family doctor in a province that has almost 10,000, and you get a sense of the scope of how much these delays are going to affect people.*

Numerous patients will be negatively impacted in a myriad of ways from the cancellation of elective procedures, prevention, and wellness programs, the closing of medical clinics, as well as numerous other services. There are numerous data showing that the death counts because of the lockdown will far exceed the death counts from COVID-19 because of these missed opportunities.

Lockdown Measures are Blunt Instruments

If you require surgery, would you prefer the surgeon to use a plastic knife to make your incisions, or would you prefer a fine, precise scalpel? Using the plastic knife may save your life if there are no other options, but it will cause collateral damage while using the scalpel will result in less harm. As scientific knowledge regarding COVID-19 increases, we should be able to fine-tune our instruments of controlling the virus. The initial drastic measures will be necessary because we simply will not have enough data on transmission. This is like using a blunt instrument in surgery because we simply do not have any better instruments available. But it causes a tremendous amount of collateral damage. As knowledge emerges, however, we should be able to evolve to more precise instruments that cause less damage.

The Collapse of Mental Health

One of the greatest collateral damages from the lockdown will be mental health. Job losses will result in financial difficulties. There will be decreased social networking and daily activities. This will result in huge spikes in domestic abuse and increased loneliness.

Loneliness is enormously detrimental to our health. Studies show it is as dangerous as smoking, alcohol addiction, and watching the news all day. People need to be aware of the dangers of loneliness and make efforts to network socially despite the need for physical distancing. The isolation will also increase alcohol and drug abuse. Many people will be treating alcohol as the fifth food group, and death rates from drug overdoses will surge.

Here is some further context to provide another reality-based perspective. In June, there will be eleven COVID-19 deaths in BC. Want to know how that number compares to that province's overdose deaths? One hundred and seventy-five. That means sixteen people will die from overdose for every person dying of COVID-19. This puts into perspective the exaggerated impact of COVID-19 deaths prominent in many people's minds, relative to deaths from other causes.

Cost of Safetyism—Are Fears Outweighing Risks?

Is the cost of safetyism mass hysteria? Will our goal of saving lives cause more despair and shortened lifespans from collateral damage? We see this problem not just in the COVID-19 response but also in the past few decades with increased coddling and over-protecting of our children, trying to keep kids in a bubble where they cannot scrape their knees or bruise their shins. Parents' excess fears of their children injuring themselves in playgrounds and trying to protect them by micromanaging their every move can result in more harm than good. One of the consequences is believed to be a rise in anxiety among the youth. Our fears are often not proportional to the risks.

Think about this question for a moment. What are you more likely to be killed by: a deer or a shark? The answer is a deer. More people are killed on the road from hitting a deer than from a shark attack. Yet no one thinks about Bambi being more deadly than Jaws. That is because there are no screaming headlines every time someone dies from hitting a deer. It is far more cringeworthy to read about death from a shark attack.

I do not ever recall any recommendations to stop driving because it "may be possible" to die in a motor vehicle accident. Nevertheless, the policies advising businesses to obsessively sterilize every nanometer of surface or temperature screening remains. Numerous scientists will speak out against these misguided policy decisions based on fear of surface transmission and optics to make people feel something is being done. Regrettably, once a policy is in place, there is often inertia to change it despite new evidence suggesting otherwise because authorities want to play it safe. Furthermore, once people have it in their heads the terrifying assumptions about surface transmission, it is difficult to undo the harm.

The panic created from these ill-advised procedures will result in many people at low risk of severe infections becoming worried sick about going to work and being around other people. Instead, they will prefer to apply for government handouts and hide in the prison of their own home, rather than exposing themselves to what they perceive to be the toxic cauldron of COVID-19 in their workplaces. They fear annihilation by stepping out of their home. Instead of the virus, what will they catch? The death of despair. More collateral damage.

The vast majority of COVID-19 transmission will be discovered to be through close contact with another infected person for extended durations, mainly in indoor settings such as household contacts, bars, and large parties. Rather than confusing people with ineffective measures, this is the message that should be emphasized to the public. Humans have extremely limited brain capacities, as is evident each time one watches parliament debates. When our brain resources are spent on unproductive policies, there is none left for effective ones. People are afraid of being harmed, but their fears end up causing more harm.

Life is full of risks. We need to weigh the balance of risk versus benefit. This concept is regularly considered in medicine when we offer treatments and tests to patients. We do not ban alcohol just because people can get addicted. The benefits of the policies must outweigh the risks. We must increase collaboration from the public through education, not horror.

Opportunity Costs

I hope you now understand that poor mandates result in harm and that benefits from these mandates must be weighed against their risks. But besides collateral damage, misguided mandates have another cost.

By spending time, energy, and resources on policies that are ineffective and impractical, it diverts those resources from measures that *are* useful, such as a focus on educating individual behavioural changes like hand washing, physical distancing, or limiting numbers of people when indoors. Perhaps it is more constructive to educate the public on reasons why they should focus on protecting those who are vulnerable instead of behaving as if they will be facing their looming day of reckoning. How about more emphasis on helpful actions like kindness and altruism, which creates positive emotions and alleviates anxiety? When people get anxious, some react with increased hostility, which leads to some of the outlandish behaviour that will be witnessed. Opportunities to educate with clear, simple positive messaging is lost when authorities insist on stoking the flames of panic.

This is the opportunity cost of poor policies. Time wasted on something is time not spent on something else. That applies to us as individuals. When we waste our energy on things that are unproductive or harmful, we are not using that energy on things that increase our mental and physical wellbeing.

Understanding collateral damage in our personal lives

Case Study 9 - Mr. and Mrs. Smith

Here is a cautionary tale of collateral damage. Mrs. Smith is a short, plump lady who moves slowly and carries on her face a permanent woeful pair of eyes. Her voice is weak and has a quality reminiscent of someone about to fall asleep. She has an uncanny ability to fixate only on the negatives. Each time I saw her, she managed to find something to focus on in her life that is not quite perfect: her grandchildren are annoying; her daughter has an unsatisfying marriage; one of her grown-up sons does not look after himself. She spent her life watching soap operas, eating poorly, and wallowing in pessimistic ruminations. Over time, this lifestyle resulted in diabetes, heart disease, osteoarthritis, and dementia.

On the other hand, her husband, Mr. Smith, is a cheerful and kind gentleman. He always wears a twinkle in his eyes and a smile on his face. He spent his life working hard at his job, consistently supporting his wife emotionally and encouraging her to adopt a more positive lifestyle, but without any success.

Mr. Smith looked forward to his retirement when he could finally have the time to explore the things he enjoyed, like travelling and spending time with friends. That's when Mrs. Smith, at age 64, experienced a stroke. Mr. Smith is now spending his retirement caring for his wife around the clock.

This is such a common story. A lot of people end up putting their lives on hold to care for their spouses, who spent years refusing to heed medical advice to adopt a healthier lifestyle.

If you do not look after yourself, you are not only hurting yourself but also those around you. That is collateral damage.

Here's the kicker. Remember, I mentioned before that our emotions are contagious? When we suffer, those around us suffer. At the workplace, for example, burnout is infectious in a team setting. This is especially common amongst professionals like doctors, nurses, lawyers, and teachers. Do we think other people do not notice that we are unhappy, cynical, and despondent? Burnout in a team setting increases the risk of burnout in other members of the team. There is a ripple effect.

We burden those around us when we do not look after ourselves. Looking at it from this perspective, not looking after ourselves is being selfish. There is *always* collateral damage when we choose to make bad choices.

Weighing Risks versus Benefits

Can our attitudes about risks vastly impact our ability to live our lives to its fullest potential?

Case Study 10 - Alfred

One of the first patients in my medical career was Alfred. The first time I saw him was about a year after he suffered a heart attack. He was a tiny kind man in his early eighties. Having lived through and survived the second world war, his eyes emanated wisdom that comes with having grown from his experiences. At the end of the first appointment he had with me, his son asked if Alfred would be allowed to go fishing.

The only experience I had with fishing was catching sunfish in the lake when I was a kid. So, I thought, why not? Catching tiny fishes with a fishing rod cannot pose any risk for his heart condition. As a young doctor, my art of inquisition was still developing.

I still remember how his face lit up like a mega-watt spotlight when I replied, "Of course, you can go fishing."

Then my heart sank when his son exclaimed, " That's wonderful! Fishing is his passion, but he has not gone since his heart attack because his cardiologist told him he is not allowed to. The cardiologist thinks it is too strenuous and risky for his heart. You have made his day!"

Why fishing can be strenuous only became apparent when, for the next four years, Alfred would regularly bring me fifteen-pound-size salmons that he caught. He eventually died peacefully in his sleep, having spent the final years of his life doing what he loved, living it to its fullest.

Case Study 11 - Stanley

Contrast that with my other patient Stanley who was seventy-two years old. He was also one of my first patients and also had a heart attack a year earlier. Stanley was of average height, frail-looking with hunched shoulders. He had a permanent furrow between his brows from years of worrying. Since his initial heart attack, he lived every day in fear of dying.

Despite my unceasing reassurances that his physical signs were good, every time he came for his appointment, he would ask: "Doctor, am I going to die?" One day I got so drained from his repeated same question that I finally said "Yes" in exasperation. He looked alarmed at the change from my usual answer until I added, "But not today. Someday you will. Someday we all will."

Stanley would do nothing and go nowhere for fear it would trigger another heart attack. He was essentially a prisoner in his own home. He insisted on playing it safe. He saw risks in every activity rather than opportunities for contentment. As a result of his fears, his wife also became a prisoner as she felt obligated to do everything for him, not leaving his side except to run errands.

Stanley also lived for another four years and died in his sleep. However, I would not consider those four years as living. They were lost years because he merely bided each day, anticipating death rather than living life. Stanley's fears were like thieves that robbed him of years of joy. Life is about more than avoiding death.

Two remarkably similar patients, yet so dissimilar because of their attitudes. Our attitudes about risks will impact our anxiety level. The angst we experience will have collateral damage. It will prevent us from experiencing the joys that are right under our noses.

The Great Gatsby famously said, "A life lived in fear is a life half lived."

To get ahead of the curve, awareness and acknowledgment are the first steps in changing the destructive behaviours.

We must recognize the collateral damage we cause others when we choose not to look after ourselves.

We must identify the opportunity costs of wasting energy on useless activities and toxic people.

We must admit to the opportunities we miss when we exaggerate our perceptions of risks. Doing this requires courage. It makes us vulnerable. To grow as human beings, we sometimes must go through vulnerability. Once we acknowledge the destructive behaviours, we must bring in self-compassion. This means forgiving ourselves.

Questions to Ponder

Who do I care about?

_____
_____
_____

Are my actions, attitudes, and habits having a negative effect on people I care about? If so, how?

_____
_____
_____

What are my perceptions about risks that will hold me back from growth and contentment?

_____
_____
_____

What are my fears of things that *can* happen which prevent me from living fully?

_____
_____
_____

What are the undesirable actions that I would like to change?

_____

_____

_____

Who am I harming with these actions besides myself?

_____

_____

_____

Action Plans

Action Plan #1

Focus on what could go right rather than wrong. Doing this repeatedly will help change your mindset to one that is built on growth rather than fear.

Action Plan #2

Determining Opportunity Costs

On the left column, write down a list of things you spend time on that is wasteful. (For example, are you spending excessive time reading everyone's Facebook posts and comments?) On the right column, write down activities that you believe are useful but feel you have no time for, such as exercise, spending time playing with your children, or seeing friends.

USEFUL ACTIVITIES I CAN'T FIND TIME FOR				
TIME SPENT ON WASTEFUL ACTIVITIES				

Reflection 9: Shooting Myself with Two Arrows

"There has been much tragedy in my life. At least half of it actually happened." ~Mark Twain

Lesson from COVID-19

AC: Do you know what the connection is between a maximum-security prisoner and the average child?

BC: Do tell.

AC: According to a recent survey of over ten countries, the average child is reported to spend less time outdoors than the average maximum-security prisoner, even before the COVID lockdown. This problem will be worsened by the policies and fears generated during the pandemic.

Even by June, many outdoor playgrounds will remain closed despite numerous science data showing children have a higher risk of illness from influenza than COVID-19 and that the risk of transmission from young children to adults is minimal, again less than influenza. Have we ever closed schools and playgrounds during the flu season?

In June 2020, an Ipsos poll of 16 countries will show that decreased exercise ranked as the #1 reason for their deteriorating health during the COVID pandemic, with anxiety being second. How do you think these top two issues are connected?

These two items both contribute to a reduced immune system, which in turn increases our chance of contracting any infection and impacts its severity. This is ironic because anything to improve our immunity is the most fundamental aspect of overcoming infectious diseases.

Exercise is also very closely related to our mental health. It is more effective than medications for preventing numerous diseases like diabetes and Alzheimer's. As icing on a cake, exercise also reduces our risk for a number of cancers, including the most common cancers that we screen for, such as colon, breast, and prostate. Good mental health, in turn, improves our immune system as well as physical health. This becomes a positive spiral upwards to awesomeness.

Wanting Control → Anxiety → Suffering

Here is the most critical aspect of the result of this poll. Both exercise and anxiety are within our control. There are many things we have no control over during the pandemic--job loss, mobility, seeing friends and family, mandates, living with difficult people, or how long the pandemic will last. That is a long list.

But why are people focused on things they have no control over and ignoring things they *do* have control over? Remember the idea of opportunity cost we discussed in the previous lesson? When we waste our energy on things that we have *no* control over, we are not directing it at things we *have* control over.

Speaking of control, what do you think will be the next two top items from the Ipsos Poll of reasons for declined health?

If you think that overeating is one of them, you are right. And insomnia is the other item. Guess what? Both items are related to anxiety. People overeat and cannot sleep when they feel anxious. Again, items within our control. What do you suppose is the one thing we have control over in every situation? Our mindset and attitude. We can increase our capacity for enhancing our attitudes and thoughts through awareness and mindfulness.

These problems are not new. Even before the COVID-19 pandemic, our society was already in a pandemic—the pandemic of anxiety. Often, anxiety comes from the fear of uncertainty. We have anxiety about our finances because we live beyond our means. We fear the negative consequences of our job performances, uncertainty about our own health, or the health of our loved ones.

These problems will simply be magnified by the COVID-19 event. Since the pandemic, many people will become fearful of living, even their regular lives, of being around others, of going to the grocery store, or taking public transit. People are living in a hyper-arousal state of fight-or-flight constantly. This state impairs our rational thinking. Our primitive lizard brain takes over, and we react to basic emotions like anger and fear. People will lash out at each other over ridiculous things, like standing five-feet distance instead of six feet while in a lineup or being asked to don masks when indoors. They will see threats looming everywhere, in every person they encounter, on every surface they touch. They will see every passerby as potential vats of lethal viruses, even from innocuous activities like walking through a park. They resort to behaving like Tarzan suffering paranoia from an acid trip.

One of the quirks of being human is our tendency to see adversity as far worse than it actually is. We anticipate the worst outcome, and we behave according to those beliefs. Fear hijacks our executive brain and triggers us to make bad decisions.

Shooting Ourselves with the Second Arrow

There is a metaphor that when a negative event occurs, we are shot by two arrows. The first arrow is the undesirable event. In this case, it is the pandemic. The resulting lockdown will cost us job loss, isolation, and financial crisis. This first arrow causes pain and suffering. The event will then be followed by a second arrow.

What is the second arrow?

Our thoughts and perspectives. "OMG, this is going to last forever. I will never see freedom again. I will lose my job. I won't be able to feed myself or my family. We will end up living under a pile of cardboard boxes under the bridge at the Don Valley Parkway, trying to make a dollar by begging strangers to let us squeegee their car windshields at traffic light intersections!!!!"

The second arrow is the suffering we inflict on ourselves when we stop exercising and start overeating and catastrophizing the effects of the pandemic on our lives. We behave as if Armageddon has befallen us, and the negative impact will be permanent and personal. Seems like the second arrow causes more suffering than the first, doesn't it?

> *"Most of what we dread comes to nothing."* ~Seneca

Our thoughts are not real. They are stories we tell ourselves, and these stories are based on our mindsets. Our thoughts affect our behaviour and our health.

Eventually, our beliefs and expectations can become a self-fulfilling prophecy.

Have you ever heard of the "nocebo" effect? You are no doubt aware of the placebo effect when a person experiences benefits from a substance that has no health benefits, simply because the person believes it will help. Well, the nocebo effect is the opposite, where a patient will experience negative effects from treatment simply because of negative expectations. For example, some patients will read the list of potential side effects listed for their medication, then experience these side effects simply by believing it will happen. That is the nocebo effect. It is an example of the second arrow.

Recognizing the second arrow helps us stay ahead of the curve

Case Study 13 - Jennifer

Let us contrast that with Jennifer when her mammogram reported some irregularity and required a biopsy. Jennifer is a petite forty-eight-year-old woman. She is friendly and normally has a sense of level-headedness. Despite being told that up to a third of screening mammograms will show irregularities, which prompts further testing, and this is in no way worrisome, she plunged into a huge panic. While waiting for the biopsy results, she was unable to sleep and eat. She required a prescription for tranquilizers to get through the week because she could not cope. I later discovered from her family member that prior to the final biopsy result, she had told her family and close friends that she was diagnosed with cancer because that is what she believed.

Her biopsy results ultimately came back normal, so she did not have cancer after all. But she behaved as if she did and tortured herself based on those false beliefs. The anxiety took her rational brain offline.

Mission Possible: Control the Controllable

Neither of these patients had any control over their diagnosis at the time, but they had control over their attitudes and responses. Control the controllable. We can cultivate the presence of mind to respond rationally to situations. It will reduce the fight or flight state, which can lead us to a path of behaviours more dangerous than the event that caused the first arrow of suffering. Our choices and perspectives on our problems determine our degree of suffering. We can reduce the agony from the second arrow through our perspectives.

I know what you are thinking: How should we reconcile the difference between adopting the perspectives of blind optimism versus reality?

Case Study 14 - Carlos

Let us look at Carlos. He is a big athletic man. Despite his large build, he is soft-spoken, always exuding a manner of authenticity. He regularly participated in training for marathons and triathlons. During a cycling mishap, he suffered a broken neck when he fell off a cliff, resulting in quadriplegia.

To say it was quite horrifying is an understatement, given he was unable to move or feel any part of his body from the neck down. Right after the accident, the doctors could not tell how much function he would be able to gain back or how permanent his injuries would be. Despite the grim situation, with the unrelenting help from his wife Anna, Carlos dedicated every moment diligently doing his exercises, keeping as positive of an outlook as he could, given the circumstances. On top of that, they worked actively to inspire and encourage other patients and families at the rehab centre he stayed at.

Rather than focusing their energy on feeling sorry for themselves and what they have lost, Carlos and Anna focused on what they could do, as well as helping others. They did not indulge in catastrophic thinking. Anna videotaped his progress so that Carlos can look back and appreciate his improvements. This gave him the encouragement to persevere. In the process, they became an inspiration to everyone around them. They developed a vision of what they wanted to achieve, even though they were fully aware of the possibility it may not be achievable.

Carlos and Anna were able to focus on what was right with him, rather than what was wrong with him. They hoped for the best but were prepared for the worst. Guess what Carlos was doing six months after his accident? He was helping other people he met during his rehab by driving *them* to their therapy appointments. Carlos and Anna were able to minimize the pain from the second arrow because of their mindsets. We all have things that are more right with us than wrong with us. We just have to see it.

Anxiety = Suffering = Second Arrow

Much of the time, the suffering we feel from the second arrow comes from our anxiety. Karate students are taught that when sparring with an opponent, you never turn your back as that exposes you to harm. The same goes for anxiety.

Anxiety is the emotion of fear. When you turn your back to the opponent of fear, avoid it, run away from it, or try to bury it, that's when you are most at risk. The more you run from it, the more it will chase you.

Our emotions live in our bodies. Over time, chronic fear destroys our bodies physically, increasing our risk of numerous stress-related conditions like heart disease, hypertension, stomach ulcers, colitis, and cancer, just to name a few.

Anxiety is wanting something that is outside of our control. We want and become attached to outcomes that are sometimes not within our control.

Mission Possible: Letting go of Attachments

This means to conquer our anxieties, we need to practice letting go of our attachment to outcomes. Instead, focus on the journey. This applies to anything from weight loss, exercise, learning a new skill, or pursuing a new career. Like Carlos did with his quadriplegic condition, dedicate your best effort, but do not get attached to the results. Letting go of attachment to the outcome means it does not have any power over us. Letting go allows us to stay ahead of the curve by reducing our suffering from the second arrow.

When you focus on the journey, you also get to live in the present. Nothing goes to waste. There is a concept called conditional happiness, the idea that we will be happy when a certain condition is met: "I'll be happy when..." People think they will be happy when they find their soulmate, get promoted, or win the lottery. By living only for the future, we miss out on all the magnificent things that are right under our noses every day, like the nice cup of coffee you drink mindlessly every morning or the time spent with the caring friend that you take for granted.

It was Jim Carrey who said, " I wish that everyone can be rich and famous so that they can see for themselves that's not the key to happiness."

Happiness is not something you strive for. The more you aim for it, the more elusive it becomes. It is like trying to reach the horizon. Happiness is not a goal but a way of life. Happiness ensues when we stop shooting ourselves with the second arrow.

> "Yesterday's the past, tomorrow the future, but today is a gift. That's why it's called the present." ~Bill Keane

Questions to Ponder

When it comes to your goals and things you strive for, ask yourself:

Am I in control of these goals, or are they in control of me? In what ways am I maintaining or giving up control?

_____

_____

_____

When you are in a situation that is distressing, ask: Is this something within my control?

_____

_____

_____

If it is outside of your control:

What are some aspects of it that are within my control? (Controlling the controllable)

_____

_____

_____

If you cannot find any aspect that is within your control, ask yourself:

How can I practice letting it go? What healthy ways can I decide to respond to it?

_____

_____

_____

In 5 years, when I look back, will this really matter? (This helps with perspective)

_____

_____

_____

When I am on my death bed, will this even matter?

_____

_____

_____

Action Plans

Action 1: Confront your fear.

Like calling out the name Voldemort in Harry Potter, you must face fear, confront it, name it. That is the only way you can conquer it.

Action 2: Cultivate indifference.

Let go of attachments to outcomes. Focus on the journey.

Action 3: Practice RAIN

This is a mindfulness technique for confronting difficult emotions.

R = Recognize. Become aware of your difficult emotion.

A = Accept/Allow. Embrace the emotion

I = Investigate. Explore the emotion. Can you name it or put a label on it? Is it sadness? Or anger? Or fear? How does it feel in the body? What thoughts come with it?

N = Nurture or Non-identify. Tell yourself it is okay to have these emotions. It is part of being human. Then observe it from a third-person point of view.

When you confront these emotions instead of running away from them, you become the one to control it, instead of it controlling you.

Reflection 10: My Own Reflection

Here we are, on the last reflection. This one is for *you* to figure out what you have learned.

For the lesson to stick, do not just think about it. Write it down. Once you write it down, it starts to take seed in the brain. That seed will grow and form roots.

Here are a few hints for musings that you may wish to explore on your own or with other people for a stimulating conversation. You may find yourself discovering qualities about these people on a deeper level.

1. Gratitude

Perhaps one reflection is we should be grateful that COVID-19 is not nearly as lethal or contagious as people feared at the beginning of the pandemic. Things would have been much worse if it were as lethal as Ebola or as contagious as measles. Gratitude makes us calmer, nicer, and appreciative of all the good that is in our lives. It allows us to let go of the need for control over things we have no control of and accept all the good and bad in life as potential gifts. This is important because research shows that gratitude not only increases our happiness and decreases our anxiety, but it also increases our life expectancy.

2. Impermanence

Certainly, you must have also thought about impermanence. Noticing we can have something one day, then without warning, everything is taken away, such as our way of life, going out for dinners with friends, or going to the gym. Knowing about impermanence makes us more appreciative of what we already have. Think about all the times when you took something for granted, be it someone or something in your life, until that person or thing is no longer part of your life. Gratitude also reminds us that just as good things are impermanent, so are bad. Bad things do not last forever. The pandemic will end.

3. Common Humanity

No doubt, you also heard the phrase numerous times, "we are all in this together."

This is common humanity. The pandemic affected every single place in the world, except Antarctica. Knowing that you are not the only one suffering is surprisingly uplifting. Everyone has their own cross to bear.

My lesson

_____

_____

_____

Questions to ask myself

_____

_____

_____

Action plans for myself

_____

_____

_____

My favourite inspirational quotes

_____

_____

_____

Epilogue

AC: As I promised in Reflection 1, I will now unveil the key that will unlock the measures which help you achieve wellness, mentally and physically. The key is getting ahead of the curve by nourishing the executive brain. When you nurture the executive, you improve your capacity for increasing your emotional intelligence. How do we do that? We do that through practicing what I have discussed repeatedly—The Three Pillars of Optimal Health: physical exercise, mindfulness, and social connection. Yes, by all means throw in healthy eating as well. These Three Pillars are like the miracles people seek, but they are not miracles. They are accessible to each and everyone of us.

BC: This will not be the last pandemic in many of our lifetimes.

Besides pandemics, there will be other challenging events in our lives which will test our emotional and physical health. However, like the countries that will be prepared and fare well during the pandemic, I am hopeful that if we consistently apply these Three Pillars, we can enhance our ability to thrive through these times and stay ahead of the curve.

AC: Absolutely. Good luck in the coming months. Now, if I can just locate my future self from after November 2020 and find out who won the U.S. election.

Suggested Readings

- Antifragile: Things that gain from disorder, *Nassim Nicholas Taleb*
- The Black Swan: The impact of the highly improbable, *Nassim Nicholas Taleb*
- Atomic Habits: An easy and proven way to build good habits and break bad ones, *James Clear*
- Thinking Fast and Slow, *Daniel Kahneman*
- Wherever You Go, There You Are: Mindfulness Meditation in Everyday Life,
  Jon Kabat-Zinn
- Mindfulness for Beginners: reclaiming the present moment...and your life,
  Jon Kabat-Zinn
- Self-Compassion: The Proven Power of Being Kind to Yourself, *Kirsten Neff*
- Blink: The power of thinking without thinking, *Malcolm Gladwell*
- Food Rules: An eater's manual, *Michael Pollan*

Acknowledgments

I have many people to thank for the development of this book. I will highlight two of them.

I wish to express my deepest gratitude to my friend Julie King, who convinced me to grow an article I wrote with the same title into this book on Health, Hope, and Happiness. Julie offered her excellent editorial talents to inspire me on the format of this book and was tenacious in her efforts to ensure that I stay on course to have this book completed.

A special thanks also for the invaluable feedback from my dear friend and colleague, Deanne Grove. Her suggestions were vital in making this book what it is. I am forever grateful for the time and effort gifted to me.

About the Author

Mabel Hsin received her medical degree from the University of Toronto. She practiced family medicine for thirty years. She is also a qualified teacher for MBSR (Mindfulness-Based Stress Reduction) program, as recognized by the University of San Diego.

Presently, in addition to her work as a keynote speaker on topics related to burnout, resilience, and health, she is the Executive Lead for Health and Wellness with Altitude HCM, developing workshops and programs for corporations on leadership and resilience.

She can be reached at DrMabelHsin.ca

Manufactured by Amazon.ca
Bolton, ON